CONFESSIONS OF A MIDNIGHT EATER

Written & Partially illustrated by
Wendy J. Dunn, M.S.
Illustration contributions by Andrew Liuzzo

ISBN 13# 9780615809359

ISBN 10# 0615809359

Printing volume #001

Printed by Create Space, An Amazon.com Company

Wendy J Dunn, d/b/a
T.R.Y. W.I.N.G.S. Press*
15 Benson Street
Jamestown, NY 14701
Phone # (716) 397-7911

* To Reach Your Mind With the Insights Needed to Grow and Succeed

"Confessions of a Midnight Eater"

Table of Contents

WHY I wrote this- and now offer it to you:

**"When you express what is raw & vulnerable,
a healing can take place in the rawness."**

- To provide a sample travelogue of feelings, situations & confessions of our personal journey of torture with our bodies & with food
- A chronological compilation; an emotional autobiography of my own obesity
- **By providing you with a working, living book that you can personally involve yourself in & elaborate upon & add to as-you-progress**
- To affirm & intensify the fact that YOU are a powerful person, capable of moving along the healing journey, and for grasping & holding onto your life's goals
- To break free from the chains that bind you away from life
- This book is a very personal & common account of four decades of self-sabotaging & suffering
- To provide you with your own guidebook for daily support, *direction* & encouragement
- To inspire you to treat yourself with empathy & compassion & know you are not alone
- **A layman's approach to clinical jargon**
- To offer you a roadmap by which you can engage your own healing journey
- **To know you are a part of a family of survivors**

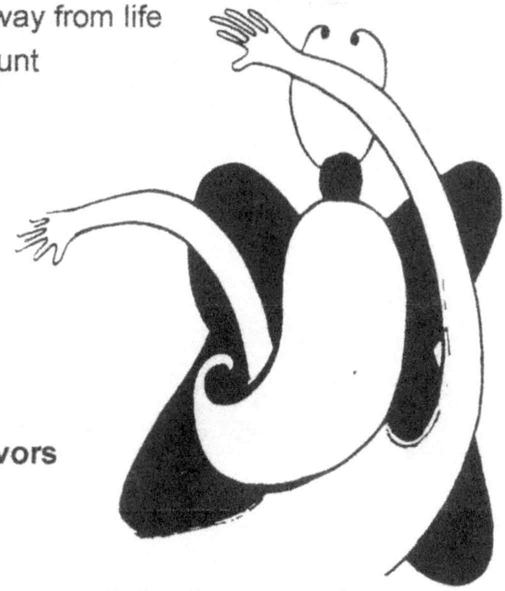

WHO should read this guidebook?

- THE OBESE & OBESE SURVIVORS : to help them get in touch with their pain, climb out from the depths of this suffering and help them move to eventual recovery; to offer them a personalized, easy to follow, down-to-earth healing journey guidebook and to help overeaters & survivors realize they are not alone
- FOR SOCIAL WORKERS: to provide a sequenced journey of true recovery to utilize along with talk therapy, while incorporating the ideas of some of today's best trauma experts, and to tackle co-occurring obesity & trauma (child abuse)
- GENERAL INQUIRERS: to increase empathy after discovering the real driver of obesity, while negating the lack of willpower as the cause; to understand obesity

About the author...

Wendy J. Dunn, M.S., has spent the last 24 years as a special education teacher, peer advocate for survivors, case manager for drug & alcohol recipients (most of whom also suffered from past child abuse), and children's mental health mobile therapist. She has earned a Bachelor of Science degree & a Master's in Education (through the emphasis on special educational emotionally challenged children).

She has spent the last 14 years as a purposeful, zealous & avid learner of trauma & child abuse: the manifestations, its clinical understandings & fortifying her belief that child abuse & trauma is indeed the root cause of over 70% of most social ills.

Wendy has gathered her portfolio of knowledge & resources through hundreds of hours of self-chosen university instruction, clinical trainings & workshops from such reputable venues as: the University of Buffalo's graduate social work program, UB's continuing educational Trauma certification program, the New York State Office of Mental Health's trauma initiative, the SIDRAN Foundation, as well as dozens of trainings held by many clinical trauma experts such as: Bessel van de kolk, Dusty Miller, Bill O'Hanlon, Pat Ogden, and Sylvia Ferentz.

She also gained first-hand knowledge of the inner sufferings of survivors from not only her own broken places, as a mother of a daughter who suffered for years, and also as a group founder & facilitator for child abuse survivors called Healing Hearts. What she has learned has been immeasurable.

Dedication

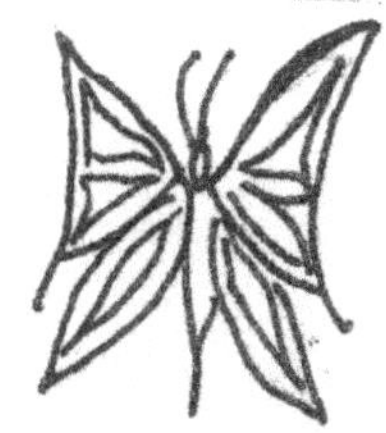

I dedicate this book to Richard L. Farr, a dear friend & fellow survivor, not only for his countless hours of my reviewing with him the book from its rough draft until the final copy, but also for his unending & enthusiastic support & encouragement.

I reviewed the book with him not just to receive accolades from a friend, but to ascertain if he could then understand what I wrote in laymen's terms; to see if it "touched him" and to discover if he could use the manual himself in his continuing healing journey. I am pleased to announce all of this was true & he is now ready to present it to his therapist to help "map out" his true trauma needs.

His accepting feedback as a survivor was immeasurable- especially at times when I felt like giving up. May he soon discover without doubt how much he is a wonderful person- and a true gift to the universe.

I also dedicate this book to all survivors; past & present; healed & healing and especially for those still suffering out in the dark.

Testimonial

I am writing this with great respect, admiration and support for Wendy J. Dunn, a woman with enormous passion & concern for social issues, the disadvantaged and survivors of child abuse. She is a woman who truly understands & fathoms how the problems of survivors originate & then manifest over the lifespan, as well as her ability to connect with the hearts of those hurting. She has strived to understand, learn & grow from her own pain & personal struggles, turning them into rays of light & hope for others to reach & obtain to transform their lives. I know, because I was one who has learned so much from her & now I understand. I look forward with great eagerness, excitement & optimism for using this book & journaling tool in my own recovery journey with my current therapist & to continue working towards personal empowerment.

- Richard L. Farr

BOOK 1:

Feeding & Fortifying

The Beast...

called compulsive overeating

WHY WE OVEREAT:

A critique of today's media & culture in fertilizing the growth of compulsive overeating & exposing the true cause of 55-70% of those who suffer morbid obesity: the dire effects of childhood abuse (sexual, physical & emotional), neglect & abandonment...

Introduction

"The Confession"

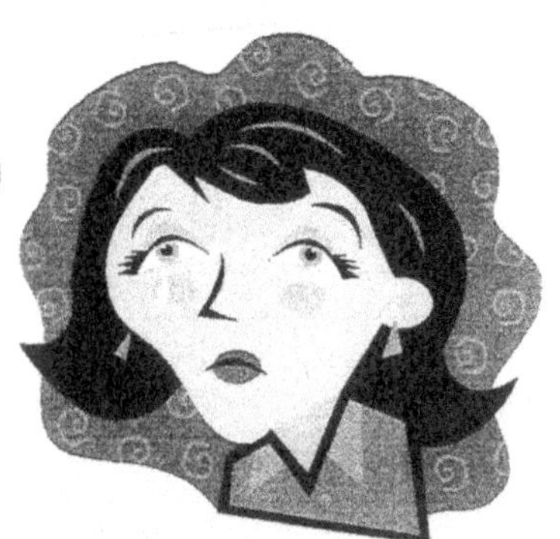

I'm a midnight eater
    A cheater in disguise.
I'll tell you I'm full,
    While I look you straight in the eyes!

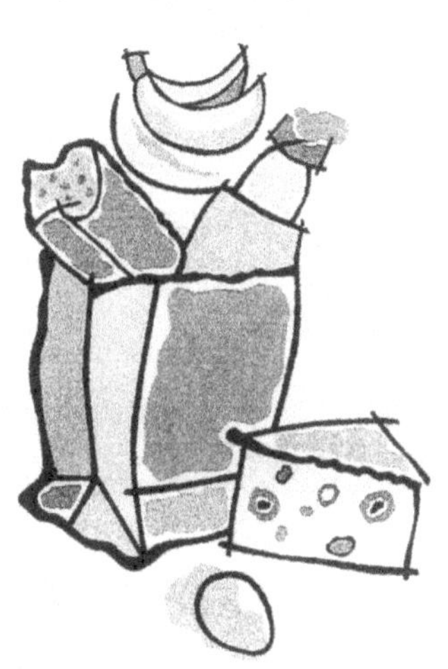

I'm a potato chipper
    A real snack food tripper!
I'll eat
all your meat
    and suck up all your cheese!

But don't stop me from eating-
    I want some more please!

Here, I'll say it:

I AM FAT!!!

Yes, I am fat! Imagine that! I admit it! I agree!

I stand guilty as charged! I'm fat and I eat too much!

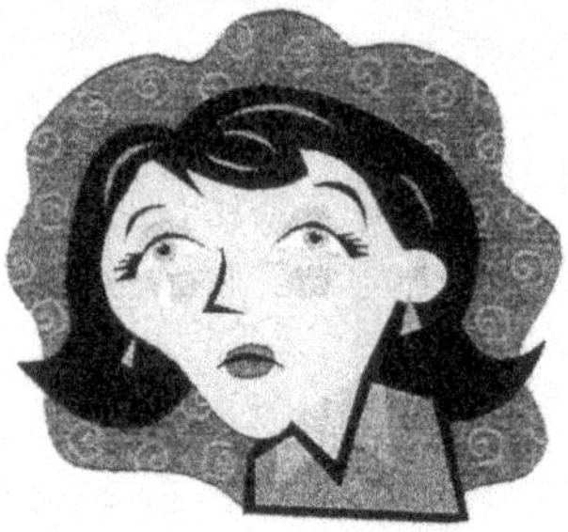

I confess!!!!!!!!!

But even though you are right about the fact of my body,

You are probably WRONG how I got into this mess.

(And that I feel so much less of a person, this, too I WILL CONFESS!)

When you're this fat, it's so much farther to get to the heart…

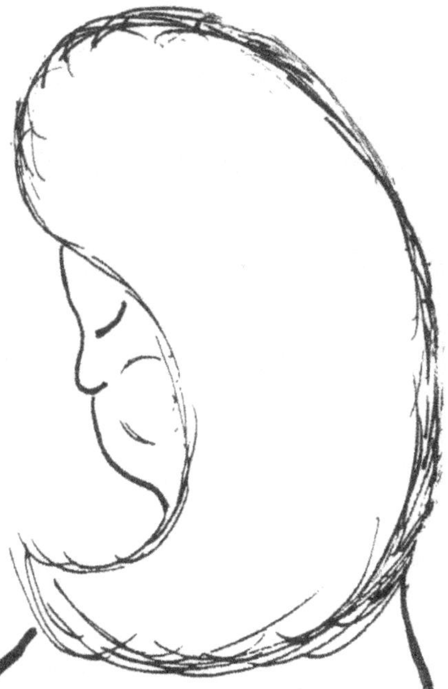

YES.

I eat too much.

There, I've said it- again.

I've admitted it!

YES.

I'm unhealthy and getting more unhealthy as....

Every minute ticks on by...

YES!

I'm tired of letting those who do not know how I tick, control my life.

(Yes, I have ALLOWED them to control me, you know...) .

I just hope my outer self can catch up to my inner soul. Yes, recovery from overeating can be multi-dimensional: I won't get better just because I eat less, but if I learn more- and then take action- of WHY I eat too much. It IS what's eating me up inside that is the key to healing my outer self.

Come on the journey with me...

Together we can grab the GPS of life and make it through the meandering maze of life and strife...

INTRODUCTION: 1993.

"Here I sit eating a sausage biscuit at the Golden Arches. 43, with no job, loads of debt, divorced, 285 pounds of fat with fears, regrets and guilt as I fathom what I have done: helping to get my almost fifteen year old daughter committed to a long-term adolescent mental facility.

My poor baby: so many tears strangling so many fears. My poor child: a victim of my own victimization. Her life's pages, a product of my painful past: my fiancé wanted more than me, you know...

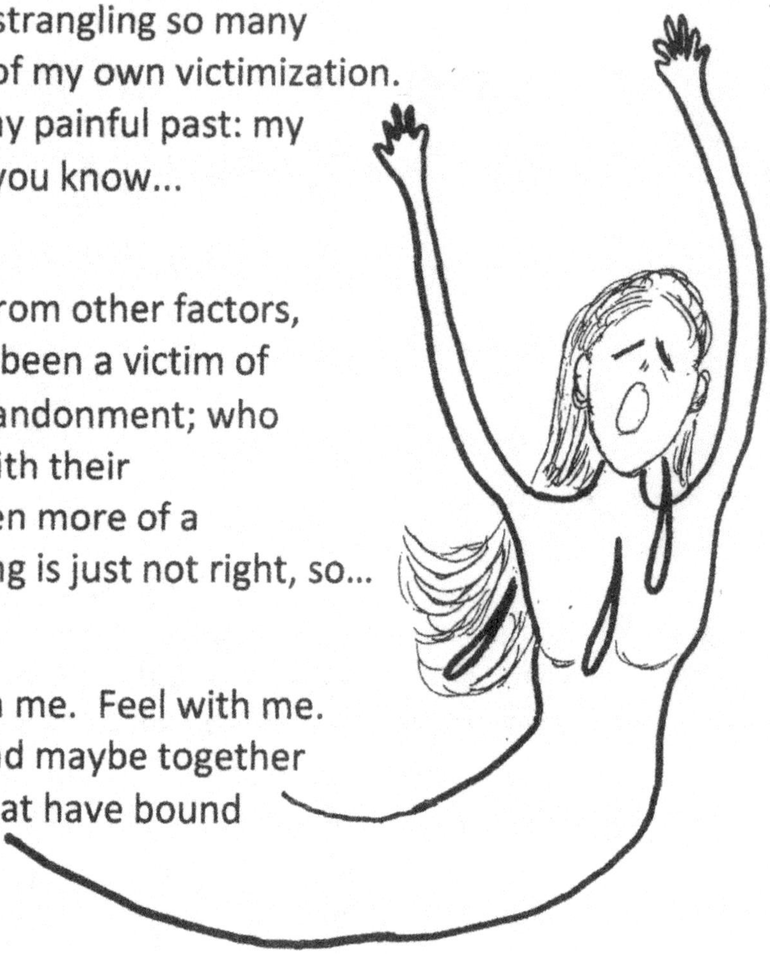

You may have become obese from other factors, but If you are anyone who has been a victim of child abuse, neglect and/or abandonment; who has witnessed personal pain with their disappointments, you have even more of a reason to realize that something is just not right, so...

Then come with me: walk with me. Feel with me. Enter my fears and my tears and maybe together we will loosen the bondages that have bound our true colors.

It's only fitting that I made this journey in time- to the pain of all my life- in spring; a time of rebirth.

Here is how I did it...

THE CAUSES OF MY OBESITY ARE MULTI-DIMENSIONAL

"The quintuple of emotional problems"

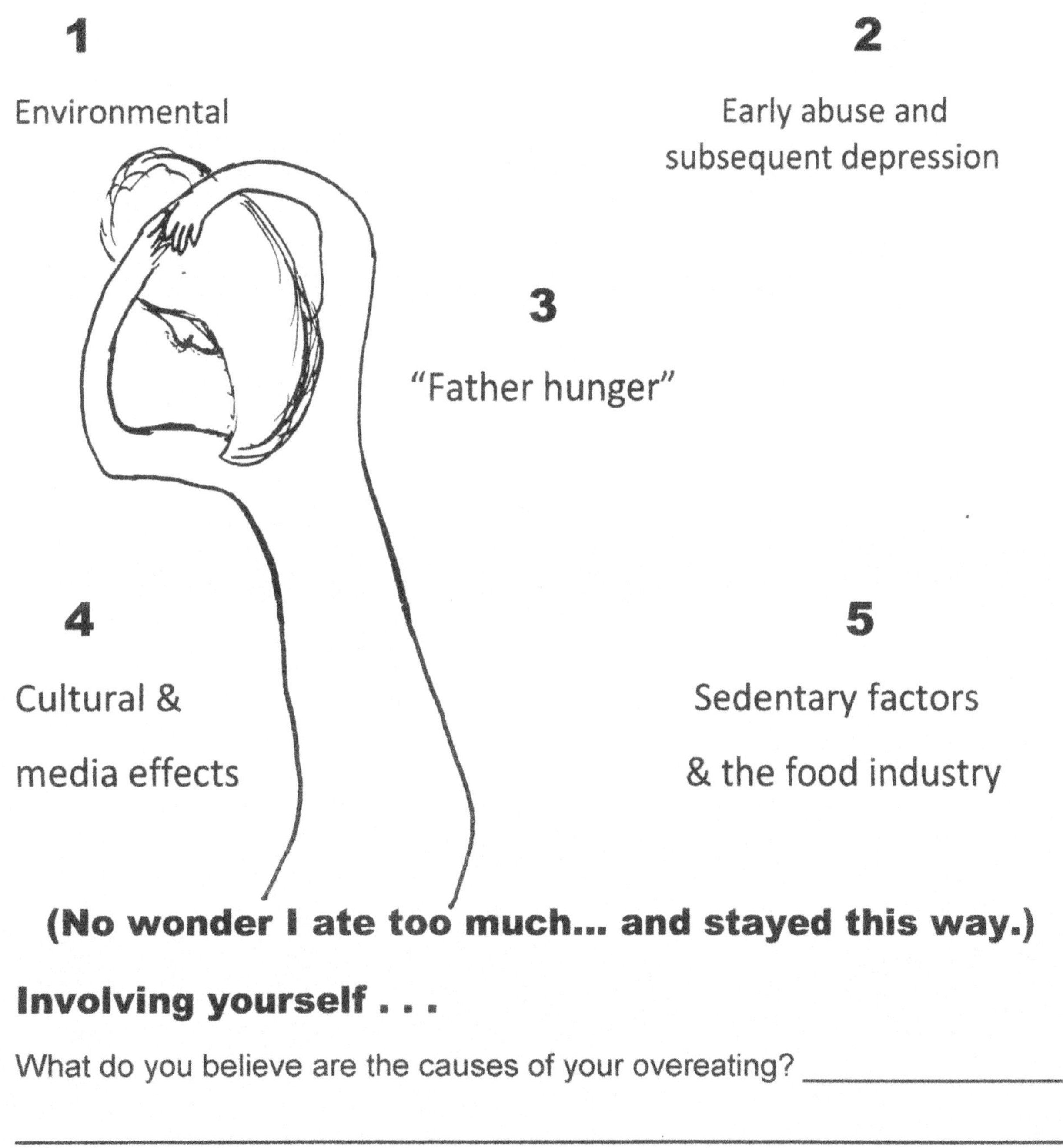

(No wonder I ate too much... and stayed this way.)

Involving yourself . . .

What do you believe are the causes of your overeating? ______________

____

33.8% of adults;

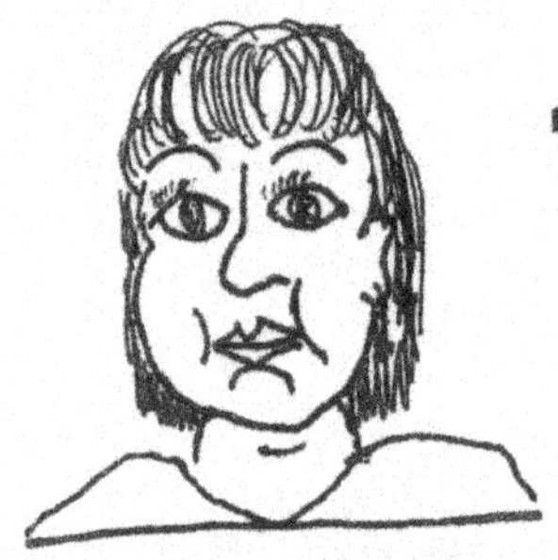

17.8% of kids

are clinically OBESE;

65% are overweight

in

America,

2011

CHAPTER 1:

The Lies That Bind:

Keeping you fat . . .

People ask me: "How are you?"

"I'm 5'4" and I'm not going to say how much I weigh!"

(Cackle, cackle.)

People laugh- with a snicker, of course.

Crack a joke, right?

Fat people are jovial, right?

(Or is it better- easier- to laugh than to cry?)

"Just lose some weight!!!"

(Or so my doctor says to solve all my problems…)

The nurse states:

"OK, you can get on the scale now!"

(I unload everything in my pockets- even a penny- hoping it will drop me down a whole pound. WOW!)

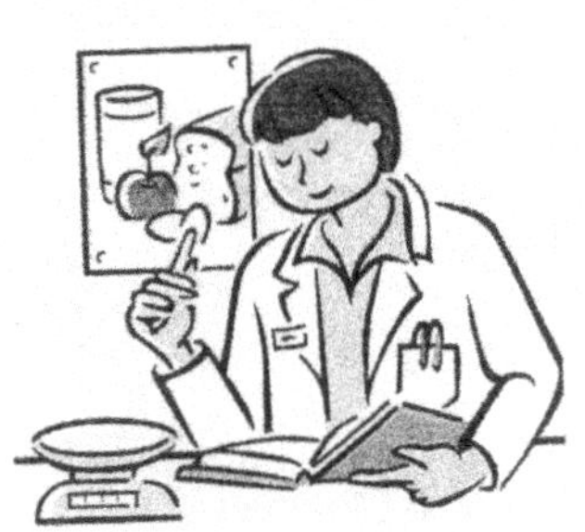

You read the dreaded numbers from the face of the scale and spit out:

"What a slob!"

"Disgusting!"

Nervously, I cracked a joke at the attending nurse. She didn't laugh, so I called myself a "dumb jerk" and dreamed of my next goodie...

There is current research which shows how many doctors treat their patients differently if they are obese...

Involving yourself . . .

Have you had similar experiences with your doctors or other health care providers? __________ Explain: ______________________________

____

____

Thin people are more...

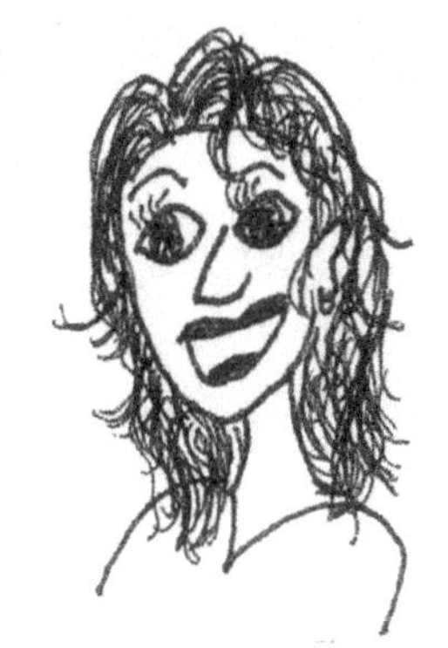

- Sexy
- Social
- Desired
- Energized
- Popular

What does being THIN mean to you?

1.______________________________
2.______________________________
3.______________________________

To be FAT means:

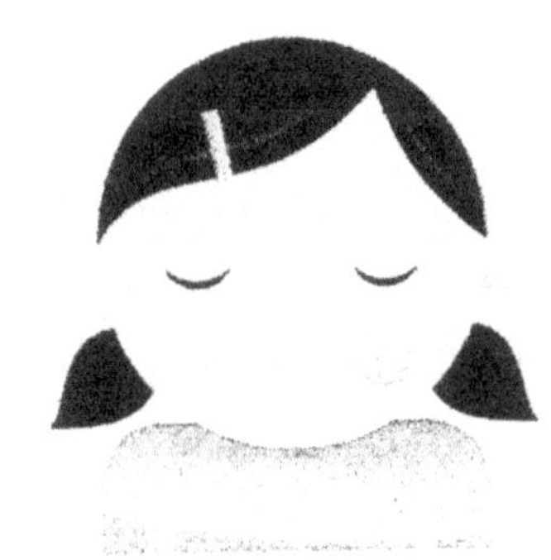

- Unhappy
- Unsexual
- "Sexless"
- Alone
- Unpopular

What does being FAT mean to you?

1.______________________________
2.______________________________
3.______________________________

My Personal description of my own overeating/obesity:

- Low self-esteem
- A sexual "turn-off"
- Men do not want me
- Often embarrassed to go out in public
- "The Stares"
- Job problems
- People mocked me out
- (Frustrated, 'caus you don't know me)
- The eyes of disgust
- (I have a right to eat, too…)
- Served bigger portions at restaurants
- Bad relationships
- Secret keeper of past abuse…

Fat albert

Withdrawn

So sad…

- (Am I bad??????)

NOW, it is your turn… (Yes, you CAN borrow from me!)

"My personal description of my overeating/obesity:"

1. ______________________________

2. ______________________________

3. ______________________________

4. ______________________________

5. ______________________________

6. ______________________________

7. ______________________________

8. ______________________________

9. ______________________________

10. ______________________________

(Now, refine your feelings below:)

______________, ______________

____

When I overate, I often felt possessed, like with an evil spirit...

...as if I had no control; that the fork or spoon strangely- and without choice- would move towards my mouth in a systematic, gorging style. Without forethought or discrimination, in and out, in and out.

Gobble! Gobble!

No need to doubt...

My possession took over and would not stop until the last cookie, or tiny broken chip in the bottom of the bag (hey, a hundred pieces equals one whole chip!).

And no one best get in my way!

I'm here to say,

Go away,

Go play!

(But, bring me another bag of Frito Lay's...)

And all the time I eat- with glassy eyes and stooped posture (better to eat, my dear!) and succumb to my compulsions, I lose my sense of self because I am not being true to myself.

Involving yourself...

1. How do you connect with this narrative? ______________________________

____

2. How do the words written make you FEEL? ___________________________

____

Don't you DARE eat: you're too fat!!!!"

When you are fat, people give you their "judging eyes" as if you're not even supposed to eat- or if you do, you best not eat more than two crackers and three carrots.

Shame on me if I'd ask for seconds or- gulp! DESSERT.

I should be spending my precious time losing weight!

Because "fatties" shouldn't eat, it's best to pretend
I am not hungry and then hide when I do eat.

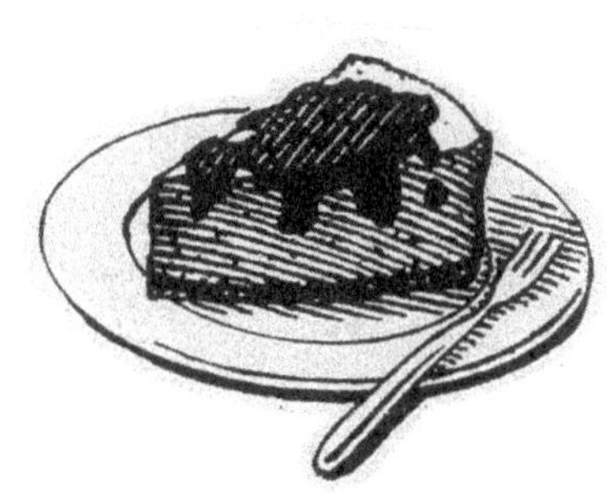

Even with people I loved,
I would sneak eat: it fed the
"yeah, I got away with it and
you'll never knew!"
(Even though I felt degraded.)

HEE! HEE! HEE!

I'll sneak so you won't see...

Then you won't ever know what's eating me.

Involving yourself . . .

1. How do you connect to this page? ______________________
____

2. How do you feel after reading this page? __________________
____

"Why did you let yourself go???"

(As if I was going someplace…)

"What happened to you???"

(Sit down for a few hours and I will tell you what happened.)

Words that cut like a knife…

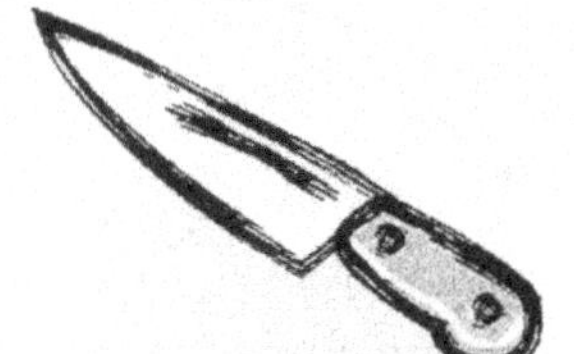

The cringe…

Nurses at the hospital emergency room moaning when a fat person enters.

Young children with their let-it-all-hang-out eyes scanning you up and down as if they have witnessed a new species.

EEoww!!! Don't touch me! Your fat may actually rub off on me and then I'll catch your disease!

There is NO such infection called fatinitis.

A fat person is more likely to be passed over for a new job.

I found myself giving up more and more social events because I felt so fat… and so unfit to do many of the activities others were doing.

Involving yourself . . .

How do you feel after reading this passage? ______________________

____

____

I'm Sorry...

For all my fat has hurt you,
for all the events I wouldn't go,
with the moods I'd stand and crow

For no running babies through the grass,
and sparkling sun,

I was too often just no fun.

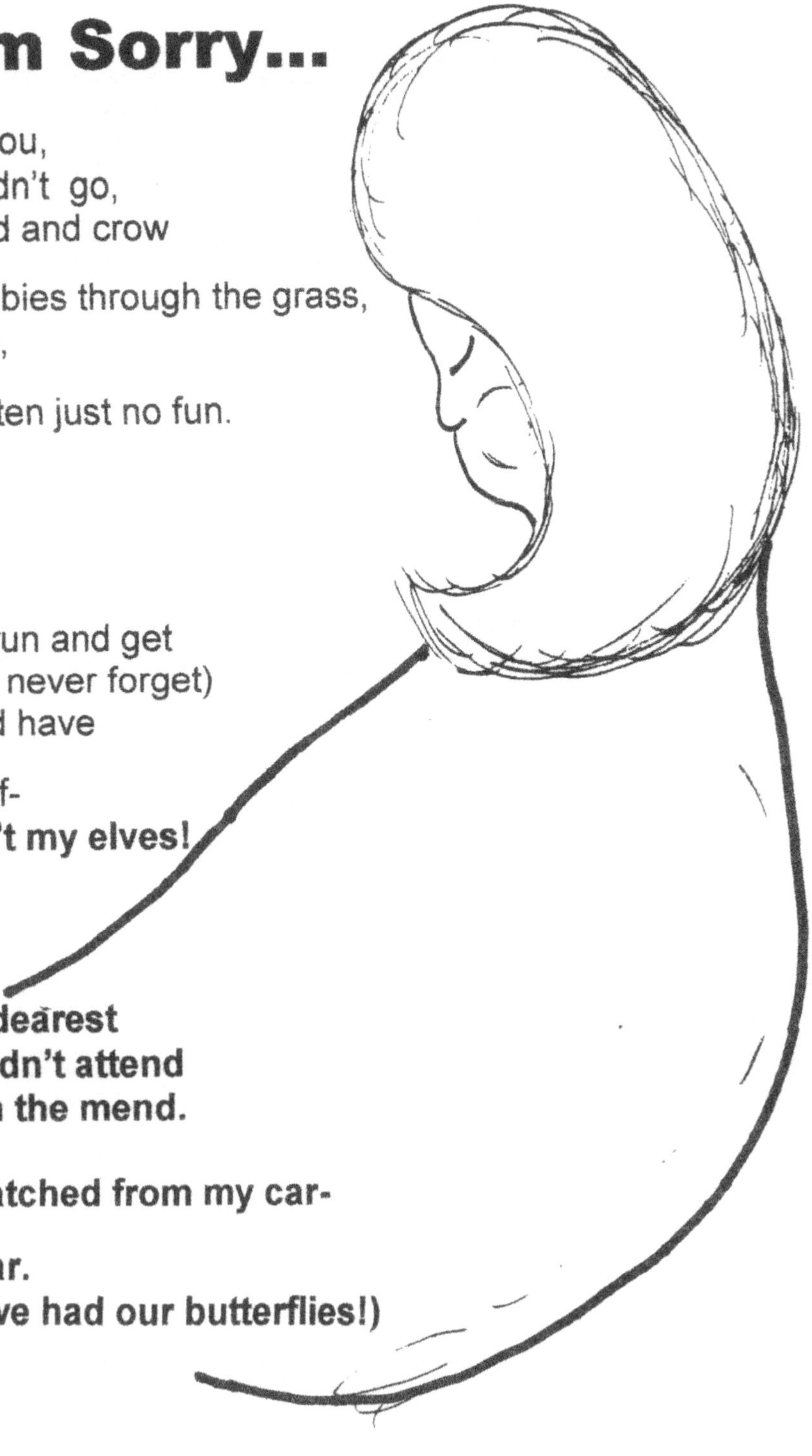

I'm sorry,
my past work mates
for all the things you'd run and get
(I waited to ask you, I'd never forget)
and do errands I should have

done myself-
you weren't my elves!

I'm sorry
my granddaughters dearest
for your meetings I didn't attend
'caus I was always on the mend.
And a picnic I'd skip
and soccer games watched from my car-

It was just too far.
(But, I am glad we had our butterflies!)

I am also sorry,

Wendy,
for cutting off my life
and living layers away from happiness. I'm such a mess!

(But I'm here to change...)

What are some things that are better fat?

1) TURKEY FOR THANKSGIVING

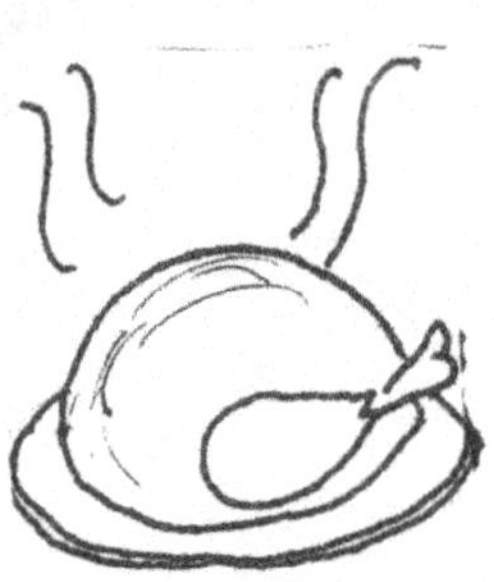

2) TIRES ON A SPORTS CAR

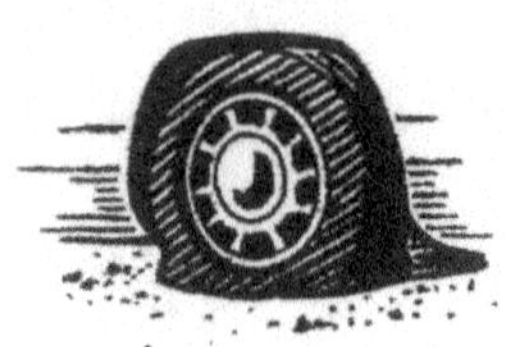

3) BUTTER OVER MARGARINE

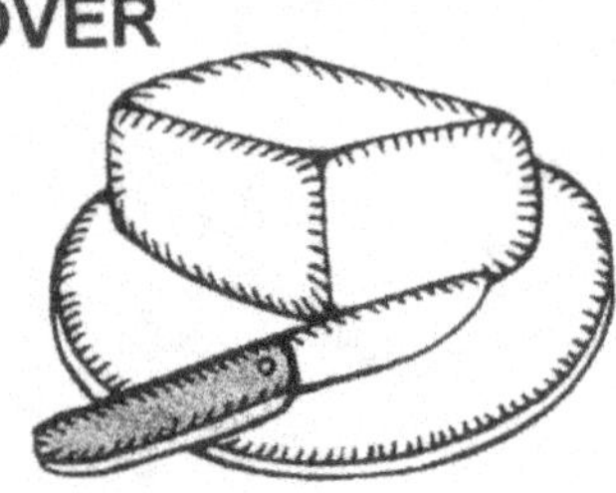

4) CHUBBY BABIES

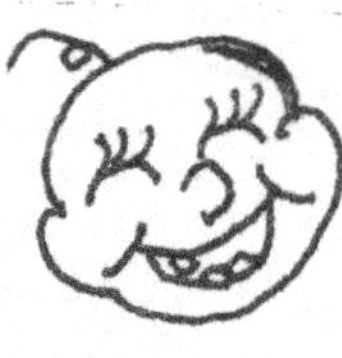

5) WHALE (their blubber)

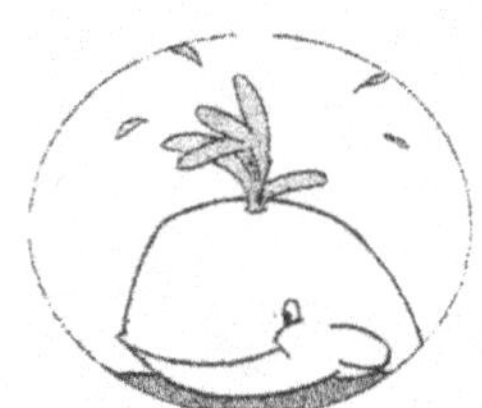

6) Eskimo

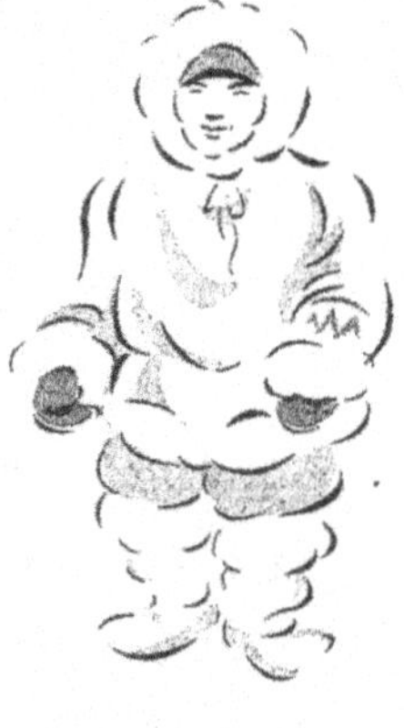

7) GOOSE-DOWN PILLOW & JACKET

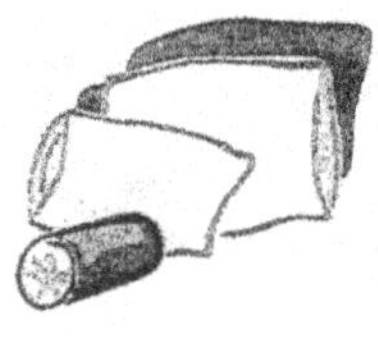

8) FAT CAT

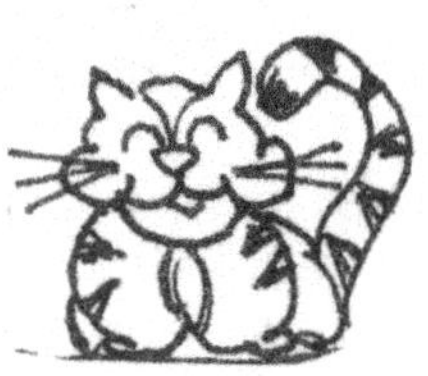

9) WIRE FOR A TIGHT WIRE WALKER

10) Almost all of the artwork depicting beautiful women of the 20th century

"Lard Ass!"

I allowed the men in my life to help paddle the boat of my despair.

When as a child, I wanted my daddy's attention, I became a tomboy. It didn't work.

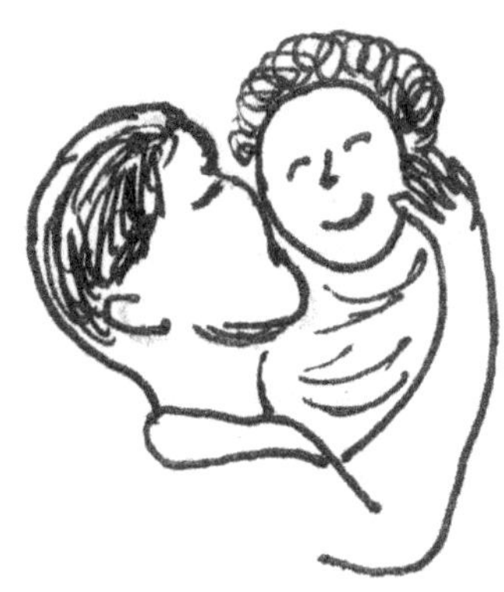

When I begged my father to let me travel with a friend to Florida when I was seventeen, I learned years later that he didn't worry about me getting with guys (in a sexual way) because I was just a LARD ASS.

When I wanted to go camping with dad and the boys, I was told I couldn't go because I was just a girl.

When I tried to end my relationship with my lover at age 20, and then accepted his welcome back (to his arms), I was warned that I might turn out like my mother (obese) if I gave up on love.

Yet another lover at age 33 advised me that IF I left him, yes, I would probably turn into my mother = FAT!

And later, I followed suit and became obese.
A SELF-FULFILLING PROPHECY.

Since I "lost the battle" in pleasing men, and unable to maintain a healthy male-female relationship, I gave up and gave them what they prophesized:

I BECAME FAT!!!!!

Involving yourself . . .

How can you identify with this narrative? ____________________________

____

____

True Confessions of a fatty...

(1) I DO care how big I have become.

(2) Many times you may have thought I was dissing you when we would meet again, but actually it was my shame of being so fat that made me run from you.

(3) Often, I appeared grouchy and you may have believed it was aimed at you. It's not. It's because I felt so crappy about myself so I may have tried to inadvertently project it onto you. I am sorry.

(4) I didn't gain this weight because I don't care.

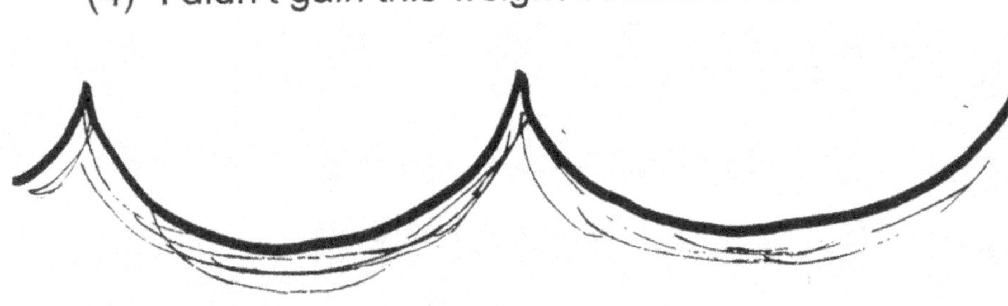

Involving yourself . . .

Do any of these statements pertain to you? ________________

Which ones? Explain your answer(s): ________________________

____

____

____

“There isn’t a word strong enough to describe what feeling fat can do to a woman.”

- Geneen Roth, page 176

The most painful part of being fat is not the binges you suffer through or the weight you gain, or how you look in those jeans that once fit.

The most powerful part is how you INTERRUPT these events and what you believe they reveal about who you are.

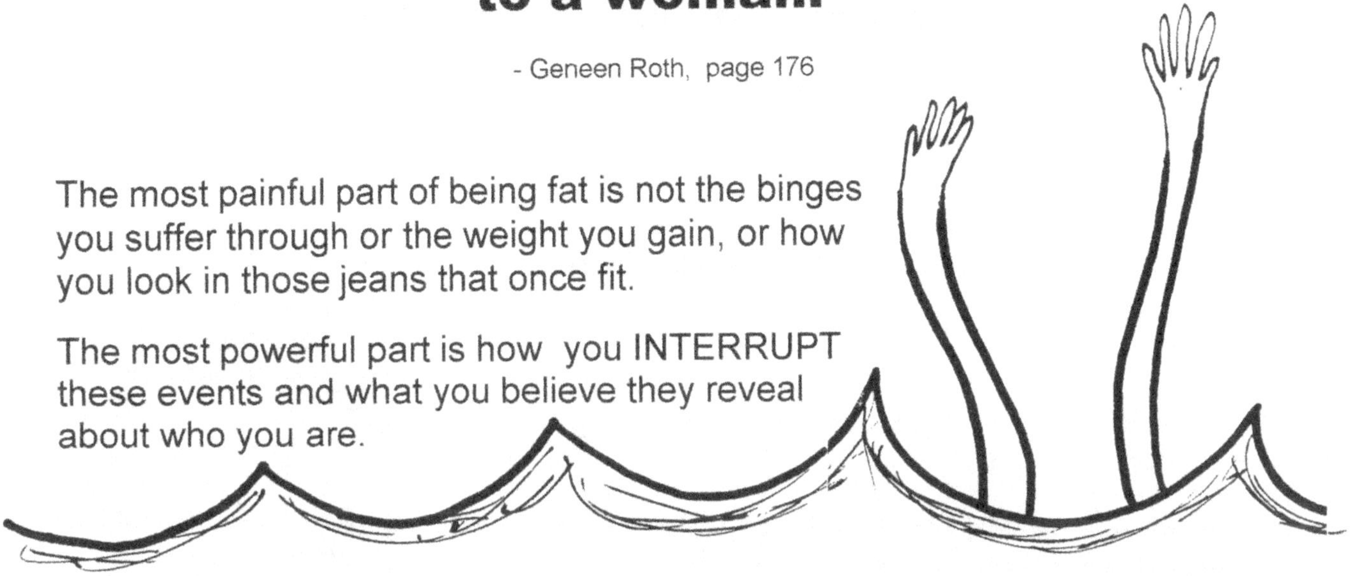

Being fat is the ultimate failure. It doesn’t matter what else I am, if I am fat, it negates all the parts.

It is not merely hate- it is a loathing. It is all-consuming and furious. It destroys all the good I may do on the way.

I compare myself to every slender woman I would come upon. I would look at my own body and feel that I was beginning to shrink.

Involving yourself...

How do you relate to this page? ______________________________

____

How do you FEEL after reading this? __________________________

____

You may say you would "die" to be thinner, but you may not actually WANT to be thinner...

Wanting to become thin becomes the eternal, perpetual need. The all-consuming important desire. It is often- and sadly- the goal by which everything else pales . . .

It becomes essentially, a love affair.

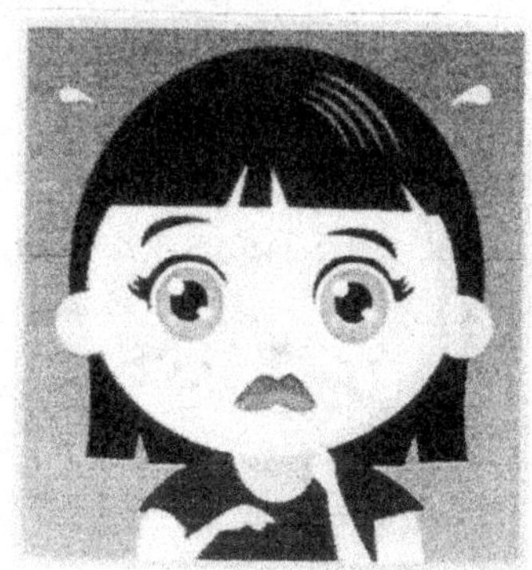

One overweight woman explained it best: "When I lost fifty pounds, I felt as if my skin had been ripped away, exposing my nerves and muscles and bones. I was raw, vulnerable, constantly afraid. "

"A year and a half later, the awkwardness and ugliness I felt at gaining back the weight was a small price to pay for the relief of knowing how to be. My weight gave me a role again; it provided me with a personality that was as familiar as an old shoe and on which I could blame every failure of my life, while I dreamed of the success I would have when I was thin again."

- **Geneen Rohn, p. 133**

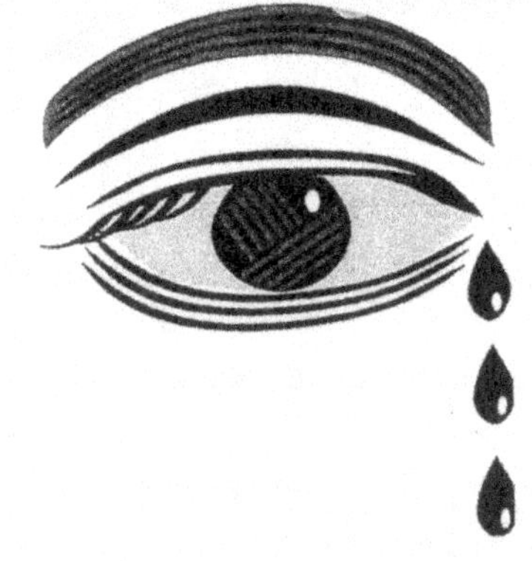

You may be scared to death
to make that journey of desires...
"Oh, if I could only be thinner!
I'd surely be a winner!!"
Or so I believed erroneously,
that a fantasy world awaited my grasp.

Maybe it's just a fantasy
to believe it is a fantasy.
Maybe this is as real as it gets.
Maybe none of this is real.

Unless you cure the pain within, you will not win the battle.

CHAPTER 2:

Diets, food, sex & other bologna

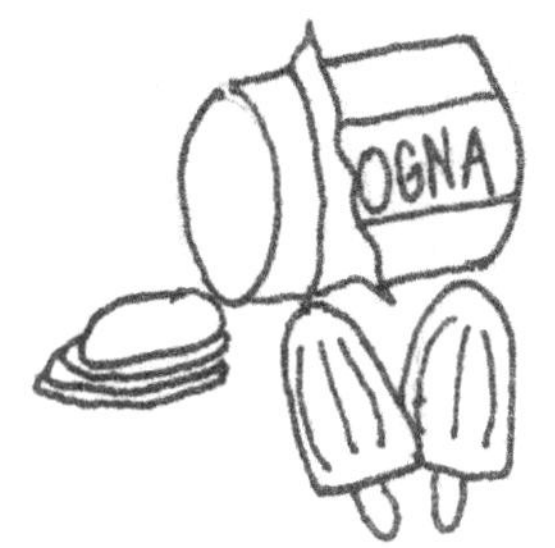

This chapter is about the continuing battle against women's LESSER-THAN-NESS & INFERIORITY.

In addition, this writing explains how weight has developed to become a powerful tool in causing women to continue fighting to make things right for their lives...

Involving yourself...

How do you relate to this introduction? ____________________________

____

____

____

AWARENESS:

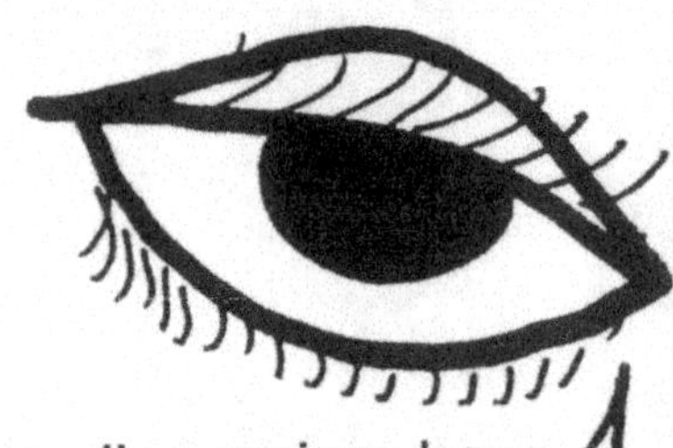

"Ann"

Ann is a woman who walked in while the author was discussing how some parents and other people down play the abilities of women.

> ***"That sounds like my father when I was a kid!"***

She remembers his startling statement to her when she showed him her high school class schedule:

"Why are YOU taking algebra?"

She also recalls how he raised her and her siblings with the thought:

"Kids, you must grow into your privileges."

((Such privileges as driving, staying out late, going to dances, etc.)

So, she kept waiting for these privileges. As a teen, she was told:

"You can't; you're a girl."

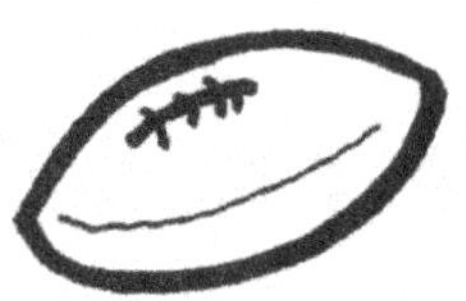

One day she told her dad:

"I'd like to play football."

Her father gasped as he pleaded:

"Shhhhhhhhhhhhhhh... don't say that in public!"

Have YOU ever had anyone make comments to you like this? IF you have, write about one of these situations. Make sure you express how this comment made you FEEL:

____

____

____

How we are brought up helps to decide how we will allow others to treat us.

GENDER-ROLE SOCIALIZATION refers to the socially learned patterns of behavior which both males and females internalize. It is the process of feeling and behaving as a male or female.

Behave!

This is a lifelong process whereby you learn the values, attitudes, and behaviors considered OK by your culture. In all societies of the world, males and females are socialized differently.

CHILDHOOD SOCIALIZATION

Your parents had a certain image of what you would be like as a boy or a girl. Most parents respond differently to boys and girls right from the beginning.

According to many researchers, girls are more apt to be pampered and cuddled. Often, independence is not fostered. Boys are more apt to be treated as developing individuals, encouraged towards independence.

There is considerable social pressure to conform and accept the way your culture wants you to act. <u>This pressure is NOT necessarily right!</u> In some situations, this coercion has caused females to ACCEPT or TOLERATE unjust or cruel behaviors by others. Becoming independent can actually HELP you to refuse to accept unacceptable acts.

Even before you were born, your GENDER-ROLE relationships were already being decided.

A scene from the 1950's musical "Carousel" demonstrates some of the feelings that parents have about bringing up sons as opposed to daughters:

A young man discovers he is to be a father. He sings about what kind of son he expects to have. The boy will be tall and tough as a tree, and no one will dare to boss him around; it will be all right for his mother to teach him manners but she mustn't make a sissy out of him. He'll be good at wrestling and will be able to herd cattle, run a riverboat, drive spikes, etc. Then the prospective father realizes, with a start, that the child may be a girl. The music changes to a gentle theme. She will have ribbons in her hair; she will be sweet and petite (like her mother) and suitors (boyfriends) will flock around her. There's a slightly discordant note, introduced with comic relief from sentimentality, when the expectant father brags that she'll be half again as bright as girls are meant to be; but then he returns to the main theme: she must be protected, and he must find enough money to raise her in a setting where she will meet the right kind of man to marry. (Maccoby and Jacklin, 1975.)

ADOLESCENT SOCIALIZATION

In most societies, boys are expected to pursue role paths that will prepare them for an occupation.

Occupational--Path

Some adolescent girls are encouraged to develop behavior patterns just to attract a suitable mate!

What occupation or goals do YOU have in mind for your life?

____

____

You may feel you have no choice but to eat- or ultimately, fall apart.

Our lack of trust with ourselves runs deep as we have been potentionally brainwashed into accepting the appearance in newspapers, TV, movies, magazines as to what we idealize our bodies becoming the battleground for a often lifelong siege.

"I treated my body like a naughty child with no control- I judged, ridiculed and tortured myself to no avail."

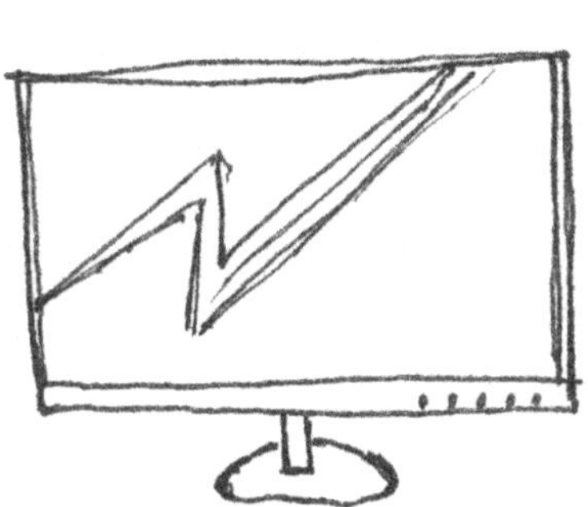

'I did not want to give up food because it was what I relied on to get me through the night even though I was miserable with my body and the overstated importance of food in my life.

'I used food to fill the empty spaces and to deal with situations or feelings I could not handle or resolve…

Involving yourself…

In what ways do you connect to this page? ______________________

____

____

____

When you buy into all of society's false images, you may just stay "STUCK IN PRETTY"

A friend of mine described her sexual abuse encounter when she was 7 years old years after she had an "encounter" with a "friend's" uncle.

"I'm sorry...

No, I didn't come here to compare tragedies with you...

I just know talking to people does help. I know because... I didn't...

I just played with my dolls and I gave them the perfect life as I retreated into make believe... that's what I did. And the likelihood is...

I've never really came out.

I've just stayed stuck in pretty.

Pretty shoes... pretty clothes... happy... bright colors.

I stayed away from problems as much as I could...I never wanted a challenging career- it would be too stressful.

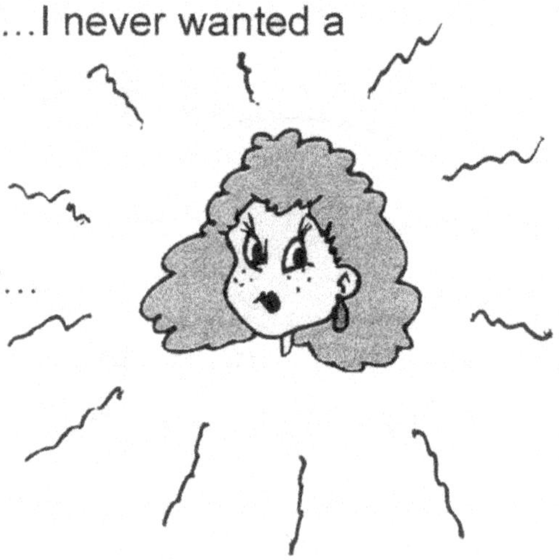

I just wanted... pretty...

happy!

You can stay locked in your house staying pretty...

And pretty soon you also will be left...

Stuck in pretty,

Stuck in pretty.

Yes, you can stay

STUCK IN PRETTY...

Are women 2nd class citizens with less than equal representation?

1. We have never had a female president

2. Less than 20% of our elected and appointed governmental representatives are women, but women make up 51% of the population. The U.S. ranks 72nd in the world in female participation in political offices-behind Rwanda and Cuba.

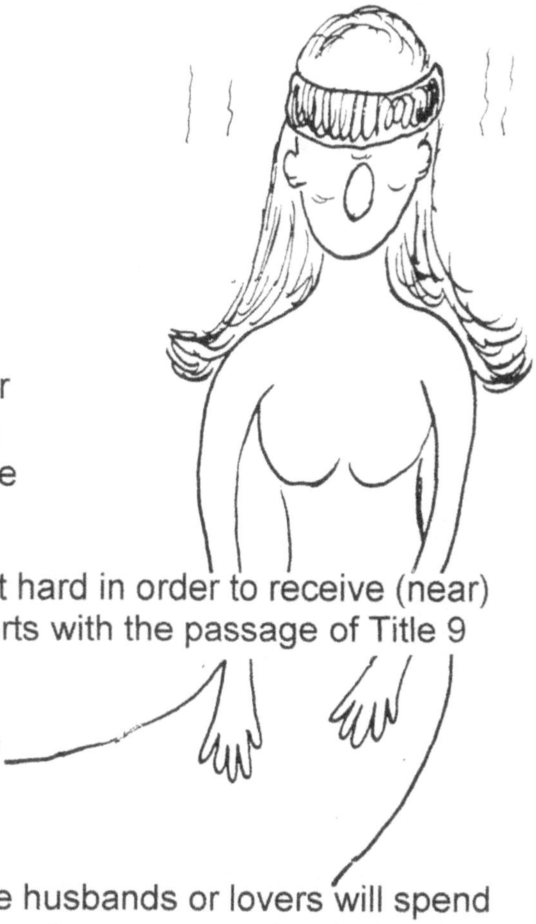

3. Before the 1850's, women could not sign contracts, own property, gain custody of their children or vote.

4. At least 80% of all sexual violence victims are girls and women.

5. Beginning in 2010, Republican federal and state representatives have written over 1,000 pieces of legislation aimed at halting or deterring women from being able to have a full voice in their reproductive choices.

6. Women and their advocates had to fight hard in order to receive (near) equality in public school and university sports with the passage of Title 9 legislation.

7. Women, especially single women, have been given the primary blame for all the social ills of their children.

8. Women convicted of murdering abusive husbands or lovers will spend approximately 10X more time in prison than when men murder their wives.

9. Women still only make 78% of what a man earns. In 2012, Republican Congressmen unanimously voted down an attempt for EQUAL PAY.

10. Women control less than 20% of U.S. businesses (CEO's and Board Chairpersons).

Sadly, with JFK's "Sputnick Challenge" to encourage both boys & girls to aspire to become scientists & mathematicians for a better world, a covert backlash began...

A popular doll came out with a new version of its beauty toy: a new edition included a weight scale stuck at 110 pounds, sporting a sign around her neck stating, "I don't do math!" (How does this make you feel?) ___________

____

____

In 1973, after a significant Congressional battle, the Women's Equal Rights Amendment went down in defeat. (Why do you think the male dominated Republican Congress prevented what had passed in ¾ of the industrialized world?) ____________

____

Female models today average 5'7" and weigh 110 pounds. In the 1950's the average model was 5'6" and weighed 145 pounds. The average women today is 145 pounds and is 5'6". (How do you feel about these facts?)

____

____

A specific Carribean island finally was hooked up with American TV in the late 1990's. Up until this time, eating disorders were unheard of. After watching 2 years of TV, 20% of the women and girls developed some degree of eating disorder. (Why do you believe this occurred?)

____

____

Does your GIRTH

really diminish your worth???

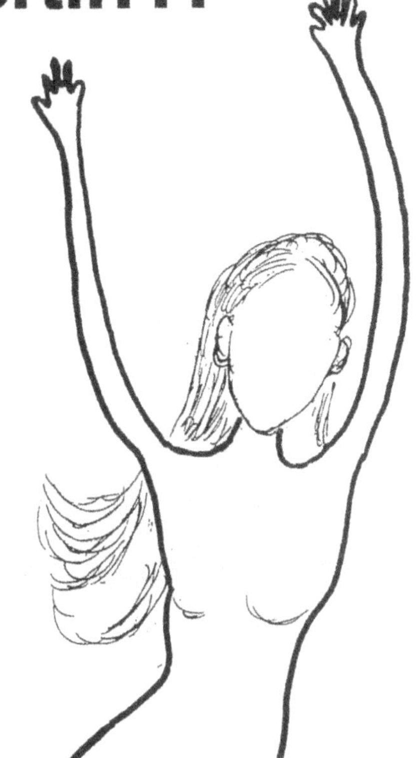

I wonder if I shall

Ever see,

Someone as FAT as Wendy.

It matters not that

Others deny,

It's how I FEEL

With my mind's

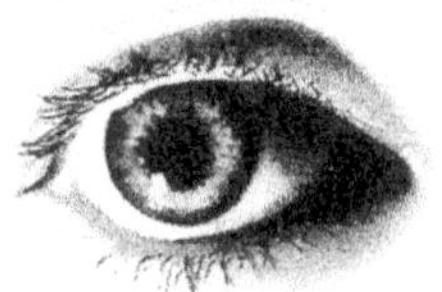

When you focus on your fat, aches and pains because you have nothing to think about, you are now limited in your activities & potential growth.

Your world may have shrunk to little beyond yourself.

What a sad state of affairs...

Involving yourself...

How has your life shrunk to little beyond yourself? ______________________

____

____

____

Am I too fat for them?

Am I pretty enough?

Are my thighs too big?

"Sadly, just when boys were starting to notice me,
I became self-conscious of the "extra layers" I wore on my bodv..."

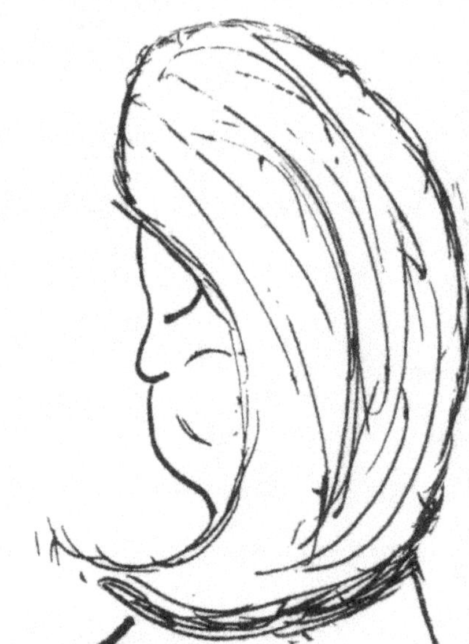

"When I got around the boys as a teenager, I could go from being a bright, intelligent, energetic young woman to a babbling, insecure little girl who was only concerned how I "stacked up" next to other girls.

Since I was chubby, I would be found farther down the pecking order of the Chosen Ones (or, the prettier, THINNER girls??)

And all the while during this time, I lost the little girl in me. The young girl who dreamed of lofty goals in life. But now the dreams were being replaced by the nightmares which proclaim: "My stomach is too fat and boys will not like it!"

I would date you if you were thinner!

(Is that the only way I can become a winner?)

Involving yourself...

How do you relate to this page? ______________________________

____

____

A girl was crying 'cause she would look fat in a bathing suit...

THE GIRL WAS SIX YEARS OLD.

Check out the pre-teen or "tween" section of girls clothes in most modern department stores and it becomes blatantly clear that these clothes insinuate beauty is found in increasingly "thinner" styles.

LOW CLEAVAGE

TIGHT JEANS FROM WAIST TO FLOOR

SEDUCTIVE SKIRTS,

SKIMPY TANK TOPS.

A question generates from deep inside:

FOR WHAT ARE THESE GIRLS DRESSING UP FOR?

In the meantime, girls are aching over their "heavy" bodies even though most of the time, their weight is normal for their height...

Notice clothing for girls & young women are increasingly tightening, allowing every inch of the body- including imperfections- to be accentuated.

In contrast, boys & young men's clothing is roomy and sometimes even baggy.

Why would anyone want to control the sexuality of women & girls???

"Control the women's sexuality & reproduction, and you can then control the women..."

In some parts of the world, today:

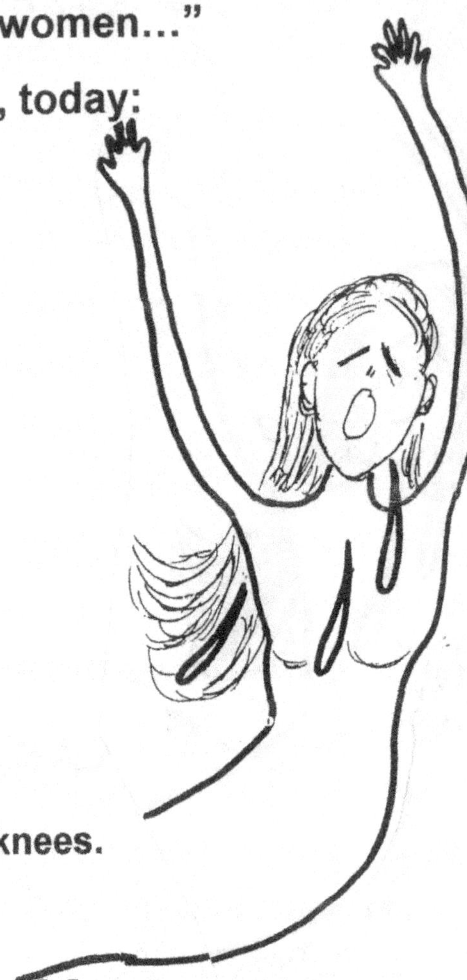

Women are told who they can marry;

Young girls have their clitoris's cut off to prevent them from becoming too sexualized;

Girls & women are enslaved as sex slaves (10 to 1 basis to males) throughout the world (including over 1 million in America);

Rape is a too common war strategy to belittle and bring the men in these countries to their knees.

Once a woman is controlled by one or another of these means, EATING DISORDERS easily follow (there is at least something she can now control with her life!)

Involving yourself...

How does this page make you FEEL after reading it? ____________________

____

____

When you allow yourself to focus mostly on your sexuality, you will then find it harder to focus on improving your life...

You will find yourself focusing on merely "getting the man" VERSUS partnering with men to make the world a better place.

If girls & women focus too heavily on their appearance, there will be little time available to challenge the patriarchal power systems in the world.

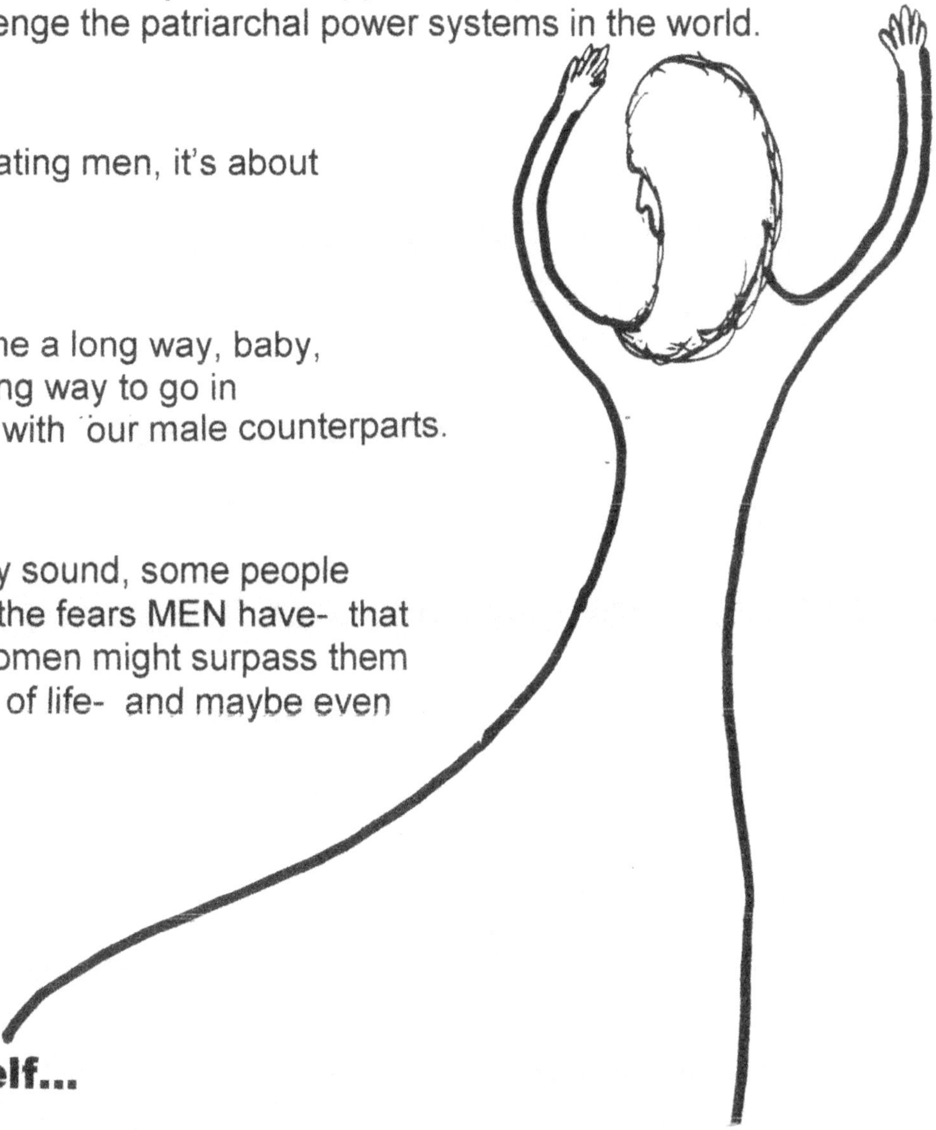

No, this is not about hating men, it's about fairness & equality.

Yes, women have come a long way, baby, but we have such a long way to go in becoming more equal with our male counterparts.

Controversial as it may sound, some people suspect it stems from the fears MEN have- that if given the chance, women might surpass them in different challenges of life- and maybe even do things better!

Involving yourself...

How do you feel about this page? ______________________________

____

____

If efforts to control women's lives & all they do in life is to work, then these women will invest little more in their lives than their sexuality.

Food and sex are close partners.

The lies that bind...

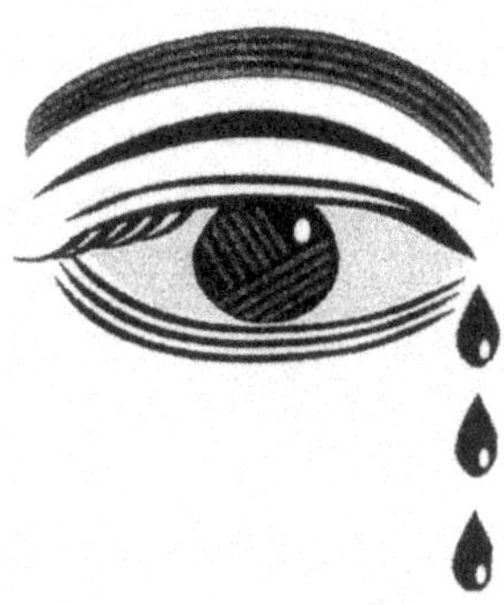

SKINNY IS SEX,
WHILE FAT IS A HEX!

In 2008, Americans spent over $50 billion on weight loss products

We are angry at fat women because we fear we will be like them...

Involving yourself...

1. How do you contribute to the myth that beauty is skin deep? ______________________________
____

2. IF you do, how could you avoid doing so? ______________________________
____
____

(lbs.)FAT (lbs.)BODY

Wide face, slanted EYES.
This accounts for all my CRIES,
There's more about me that I want to CHANGE,
My whole body is what I wanna REARRANGE,
I hate my wide HIPS,
And I can't stand my crooked LIPS,
Nappy HAIR,
All guys do is STARE,
At the way my fat body looks when I WALK,
I don't like the sound of my voice when I TALK,
When I SMILE,
I wish it would be WORTHWHILE,
But all I can do is wish for a new BODY,
I truly do despise the way I am STACKED,
It makes me so desperately, god damn SICK.

- **A 17 year old moderately obese child abuse survivor**

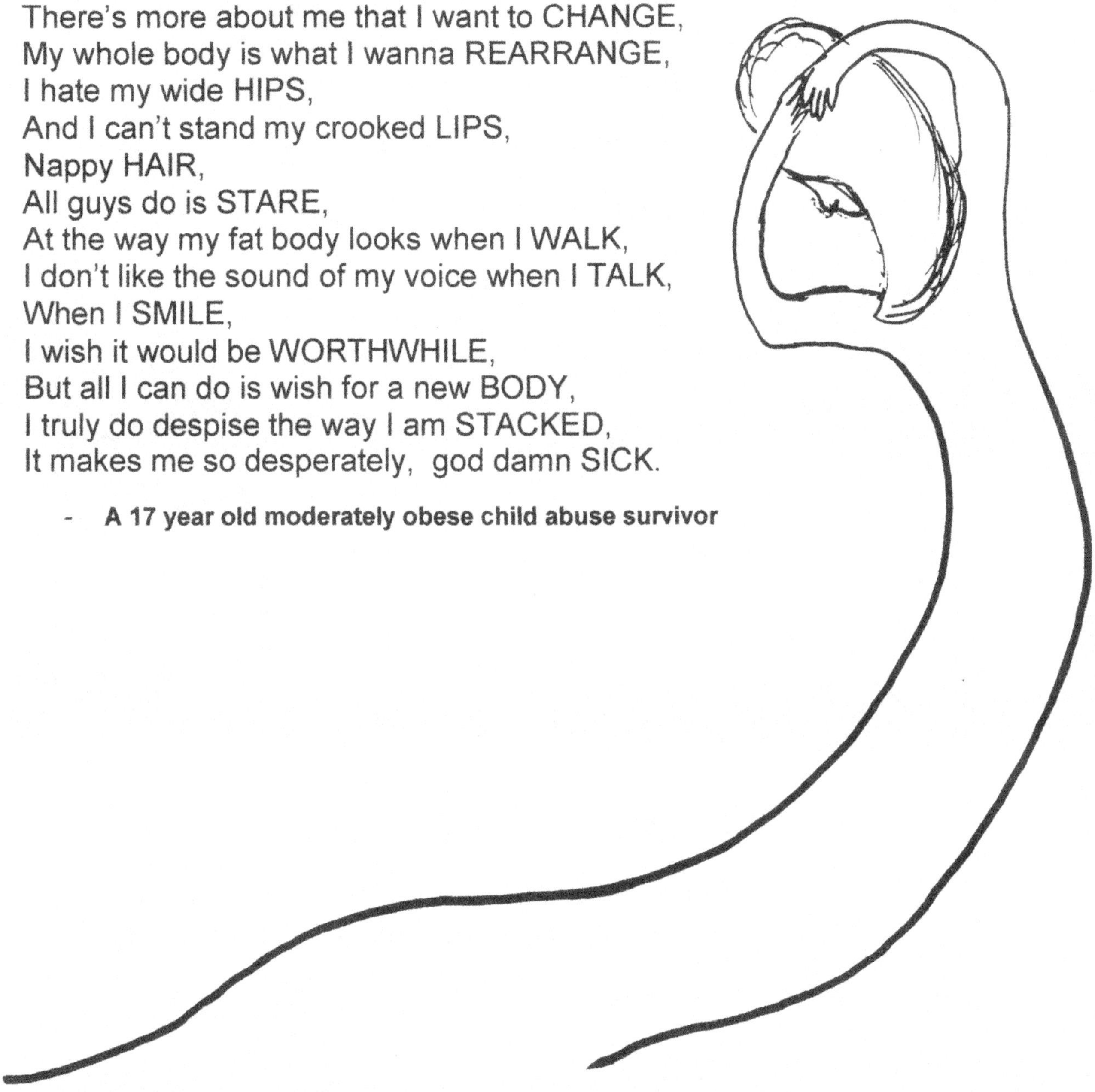

Involving yourself...

How does this poem make you FEEL? ______________________________

____

____

Generally speaking, restaurants in America serve portions 25% larger than in Europe.

Most U.S. restaurants' servings are AT LEAST double the normal serving size as recommended by the F.D.A.

Obesity is not a significant problem in mainstream Europe.

FAT is the main flavor; the main attraction.

The U.S. food industry spends billions lobbying for their entrenched positions to keep from legislating positive changes to our eating habits.

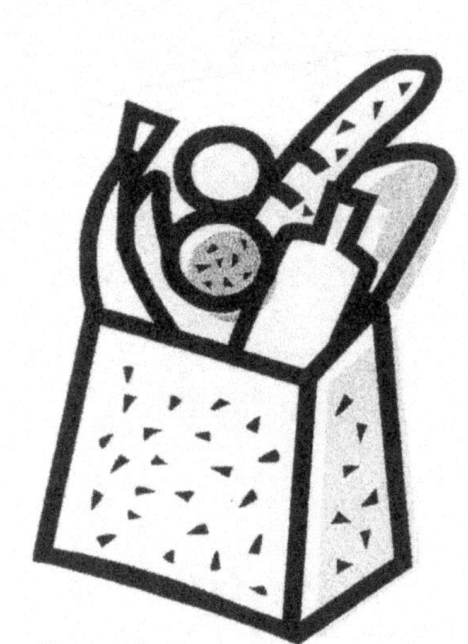

In the same year that First Lady Michelle Obama advocated for healthier school lunches to help combat against childhood obesity, the frozen food industry successfully lobbied the FDA stating that PIZZA and FRENCH FRIES are now considered acceptable VEGETABLES!!

French public schools hire chefs to prepare fresh, wholesome meals for their children.

"I want more & more!"

There is a growing- and quite secretive, multi-billion dollar food additive industry creating concoctions added to the processed & fast food industry, which literally could cause you to crave the food offerings, which then creates greater profits for these food companies.

Involving yourself...

How does this make you FEEL? ______________________________

____

____

____

The Diet Culture...

"Women have spent years trying to slice away what makes our bodies womanly: the roundness, the lushness, and we have sliced our spirits instead. We've listened for so long to what they- our parents, our doctors, our lovers, our fashion moguls, our Hollywood directors- decide is attractive that we've lost our own voices. We don't know who we are anymore."

- GENEEN ROTH, page 216

In our culture, women use their bodies as the battleground. Women's voices may not always be heard, but their bodies will speak out-

Loud and clear.

Fat or thin.

Failure or success.

Incomplete vs Complete.

Why diets do not work:

START HERE:

LOW SELF-ACCEPTANCE

WEIGHT IS THE PROBLEM

STRUCTURED DIET

(good vs. bad foods)

LOWER SELF-ACCEPTANCE

FEEL DEPRIVED

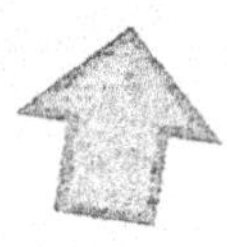

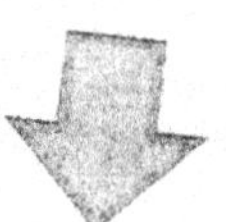

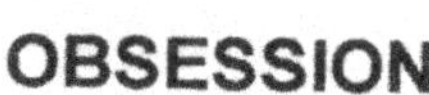

WEIGHT GAIN

"STRICTER DIET"

OBSESSION

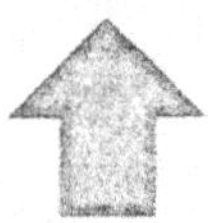

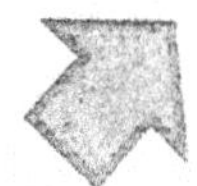

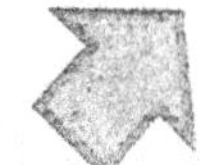

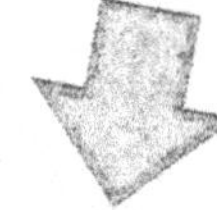

GIVE UP

GUILT

(out of control)

BINGE

- forbidden foods
- large amounts
- anxiety relief

END-POINT OVERWEIGHT

(no self-trust, low self-esteem,

Always looking for a better diet;

Angry & defeated)

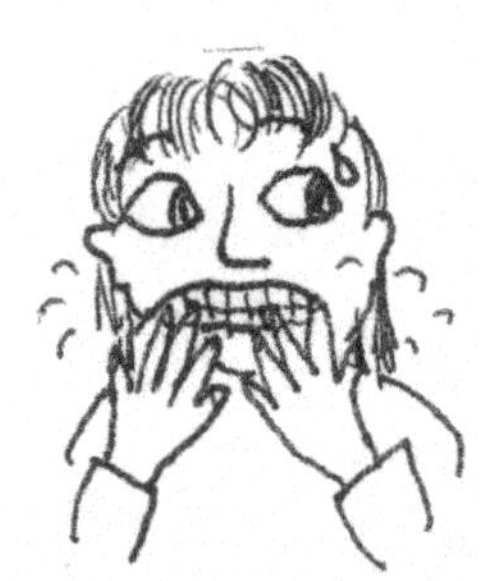

Dump the diet...

Strict diets do not work. Too often, they become inhumanly restrictive, since they are based on deprevation.

75-90% of people who lose 40 pounds or more will regain the weight lost within two years.

(John Foreyt, psychologist; Baylor College of Medicine, 2011)

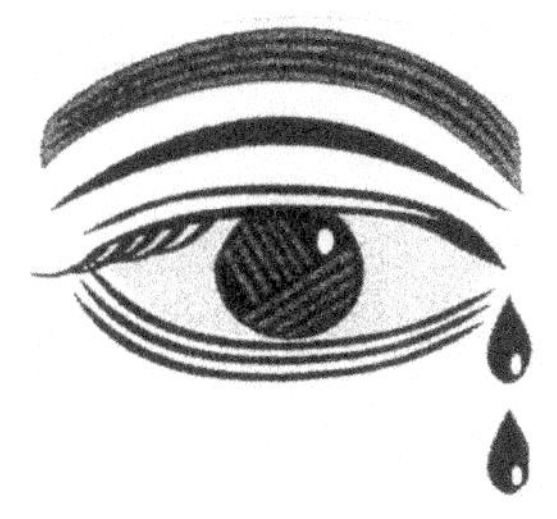

On any given day, 25% of Americans are on a diet.

The myths of the diet industry:

1. "Someday, you will find just the right diet!"

(Almost all long-term diets will fizzle out.)

2. "Follow your ideal weight on the weight chart."

(No one has the same body size & bone density as others.)

3. "Never quit dieting, because you could gain too much weight."

(Dropped metabolism and your body craves to re-establish your natural weight.)

4. "Lose weight and you will live longer."

(There is new research that proclaims this is true only for the morbidly obese.)

Involving yourself...

What do you think about this page? ______________________________

____

____

____

Drastic measures...

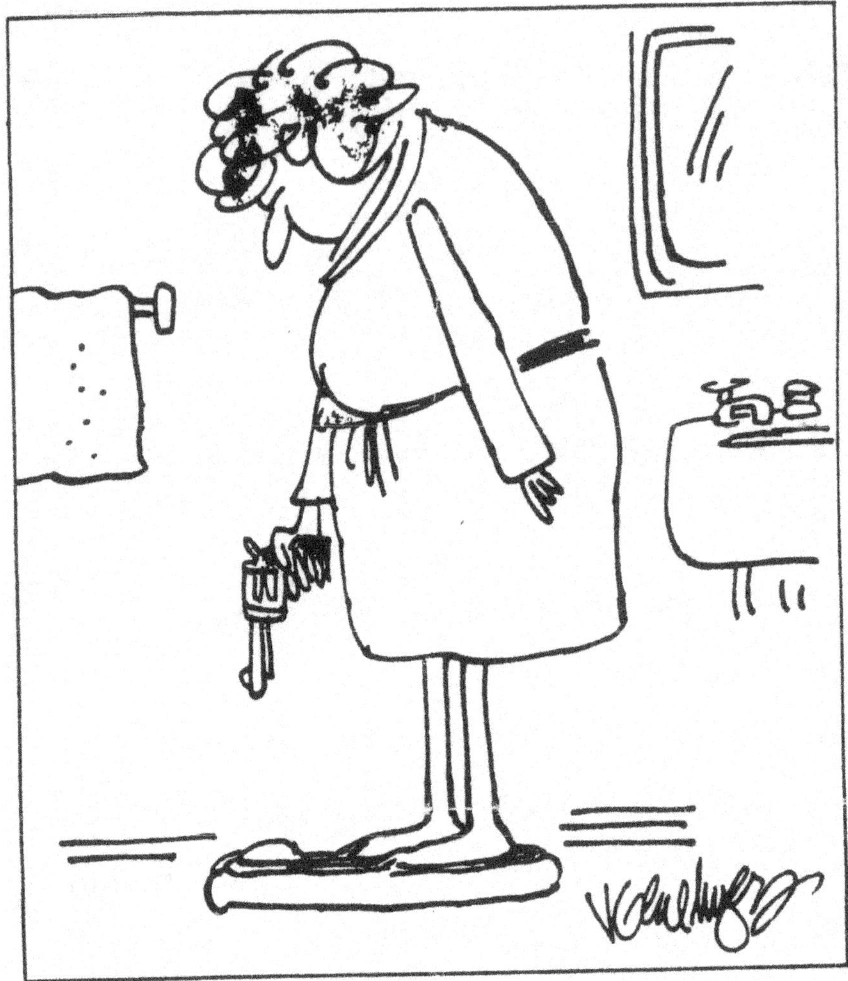

(I am still looking for the source of this picture and would LOVE to give credit to it. WRITE ME!)

I feel so odd
So out of place
Two seats I could replace!

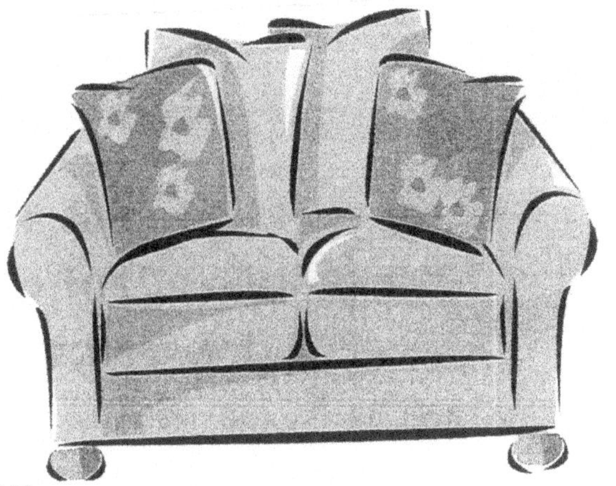

Don't notice me!
I did not gain this weight
to gain attention
but to keep you out...

Outside is what I feel.
What IS really real?

It is socially acceptable to diet & complain about your weight- but NOT okay to feel good about yourself & eating what you want...

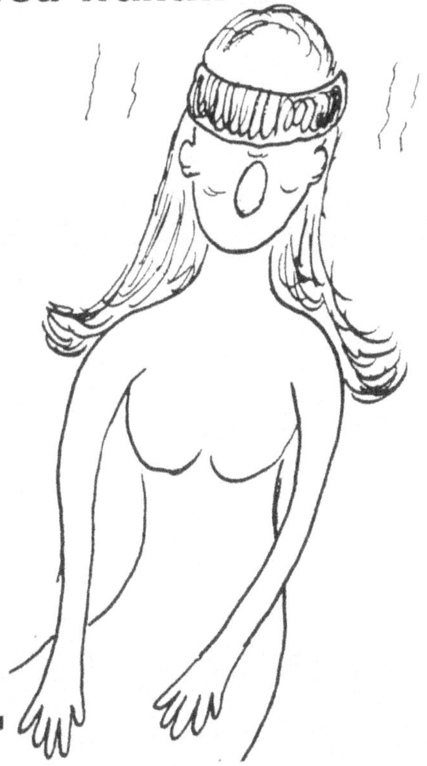

On behalf of all men I apologize.

(Spoken by a male sympathizer of the damage done by women's eating disorders, as announced by Kathryn Sylva & Robin Lasser, "Eating Disorders in a Disordered Culture")

A warm chocolate brownie is a sorry excuse for a warm embrace . . .

Sneaky eating became a sick little game I used to distance- and supposedly protect- myself from life.

When you sneak and pretend in front of others you are sneaking and pretending to yourself.

If you feel you are too disgusting to eat in front of others, then you feel you must hide your eating- and hide yourself.

If you send undercover the soft, vulnerable, human parts of yourself, you cut yourself off from what you want and need the most: love and relationships.

Likewise, you can assuage your fears of intimacy by eating.

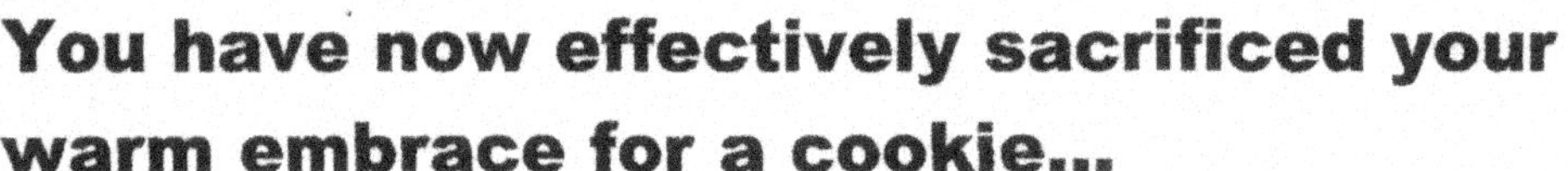

You have now effectively sacrificed your warm embrace for a cookie...

When you spend your life wanting, you never get down to the task of living.

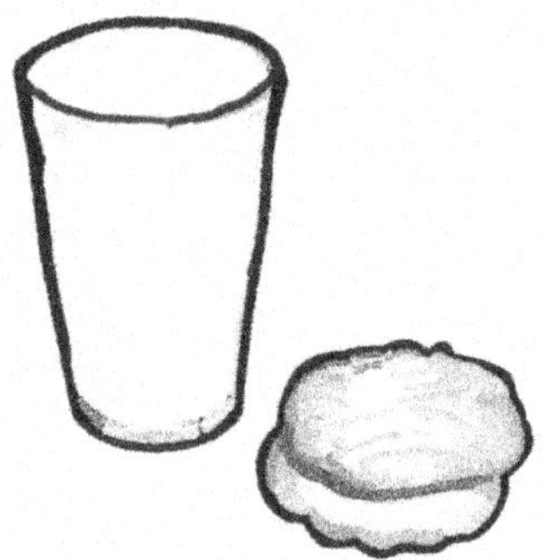

<u>Involving yourself . . .</u>

Do you ever feel like this page has expressed? _______ If so, explain:

____

"I fed a negative mindset that I was a failure; that I couldn't do anything right, so what's the use: I MIGHT AS WELL EAT!!!

So, I ate..."

The obese may say:

"I feel I shouldn't be allowed to eat fattening food."

Not allowed?

If you do eat, you feel like you're breaking a law.

"When I give myself what I needed or wanted,
I felt I was doing something wrong."

"I felt like a crook in the middle of the night, sneaking goodies behind other's backs."

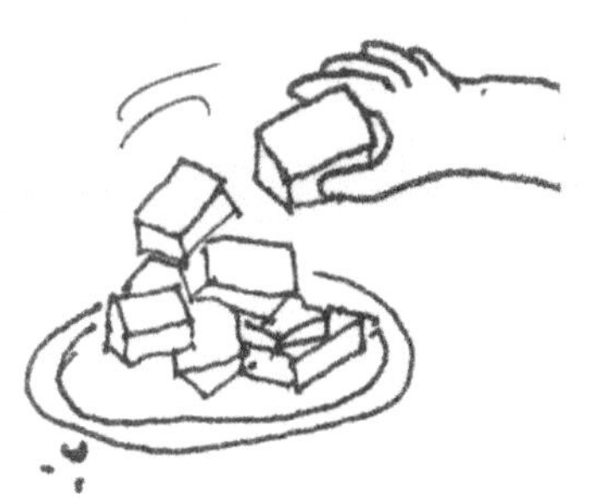

Unfortunately, sometimes the urgency of wanting relief from the pain or bad feelings is more powerful than the decision to eat or not eat 5 brownies...

Involving yourself...

How do you connect with this page? ______________________________

____

____

How do you FEEL about this page? ______________________________

____

____

CHAPTER 3:

FAIR GAME:

The bullying of the obese

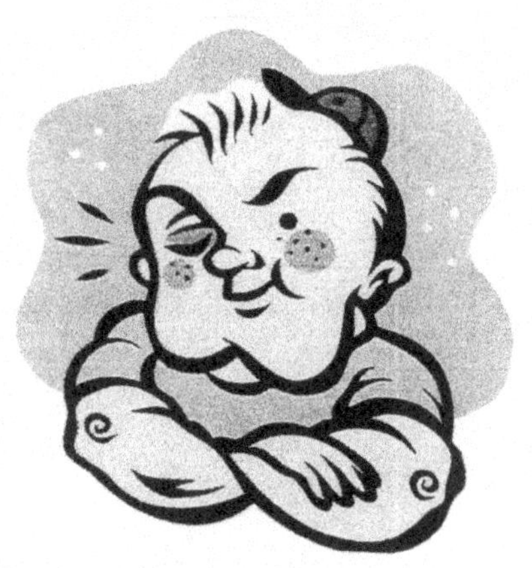

Don't shake your head!

I KNOW that I am fat-

Don't point your finger!

I certainly won't linger

'round you anymore

'caus there is too much scorn

Shooting from your eyes!

I will stay away from you!

If I touch you

You'll catch my germs

And your body will grow

With the 'disease'

That I carry...

Involving yourself...

How does this make you feel? ______________________________

____

According to a September 21, 2011 AP-MTV poll, the group of people who get picked on the most are those who are overweight.

47% of those polled feel it is appropriate to intentionally hurt the obese over other normally inclusive discriminated groups (such as African Americans, gays, and the sexuality of women).

Those 47% say their comments are meant to sting.

In contrast, the discriminatory statements of other bullied groups are not seen as being intentionally hurtful, as with the obese. Instead, other remarks are often seen as jokes and even funny.

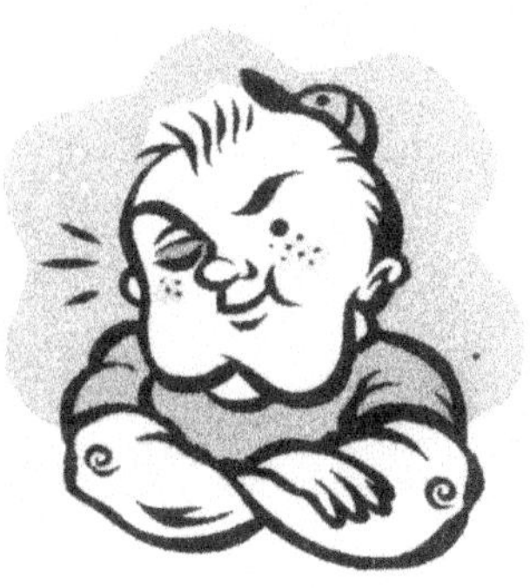

Involving yourself...

1. Have you ever been bullied in such a fashion? ______________

2. Why do you feel it is okay for some people to be mean to other people? ____
____
____

It's okay to crack a joke about fat people...

Steve Breen / *San Diego Union-Tribune* 2006

WHO SAYS OUR KIDS DON'T EXERCISE?

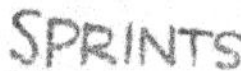

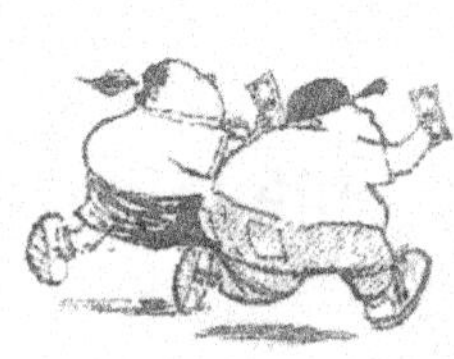

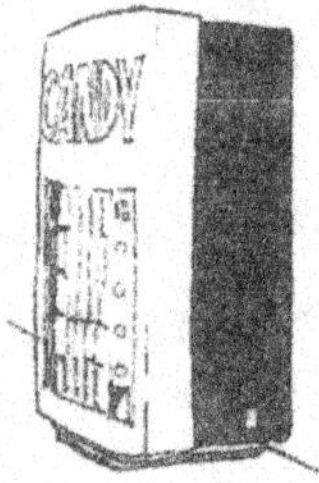

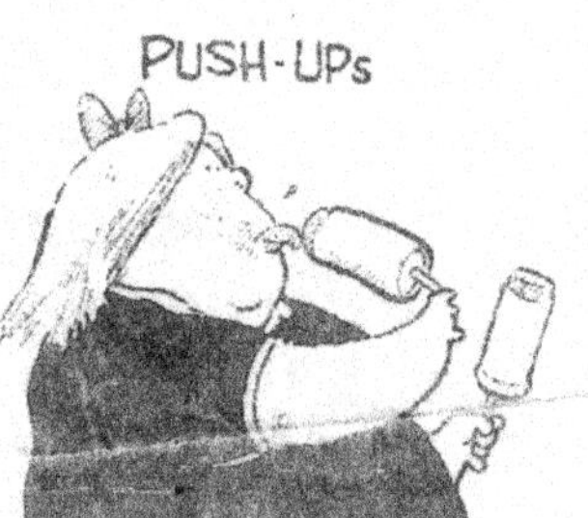

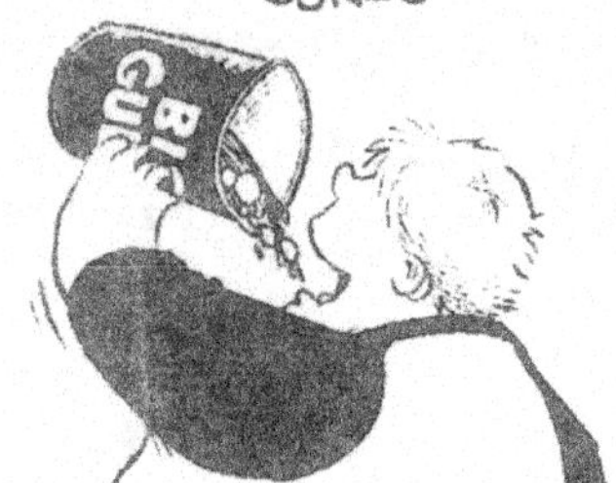

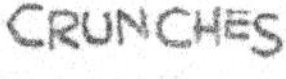

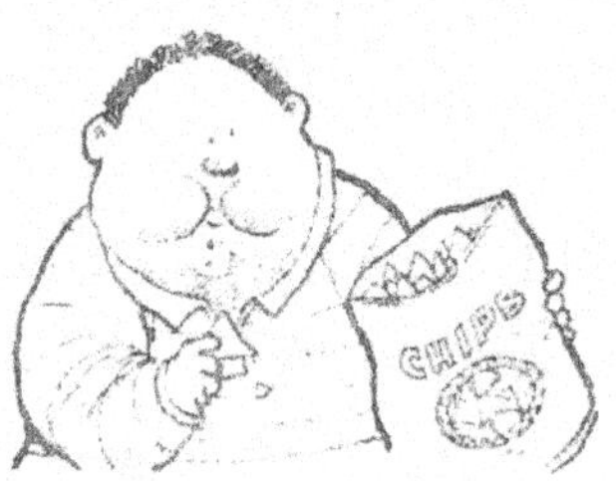

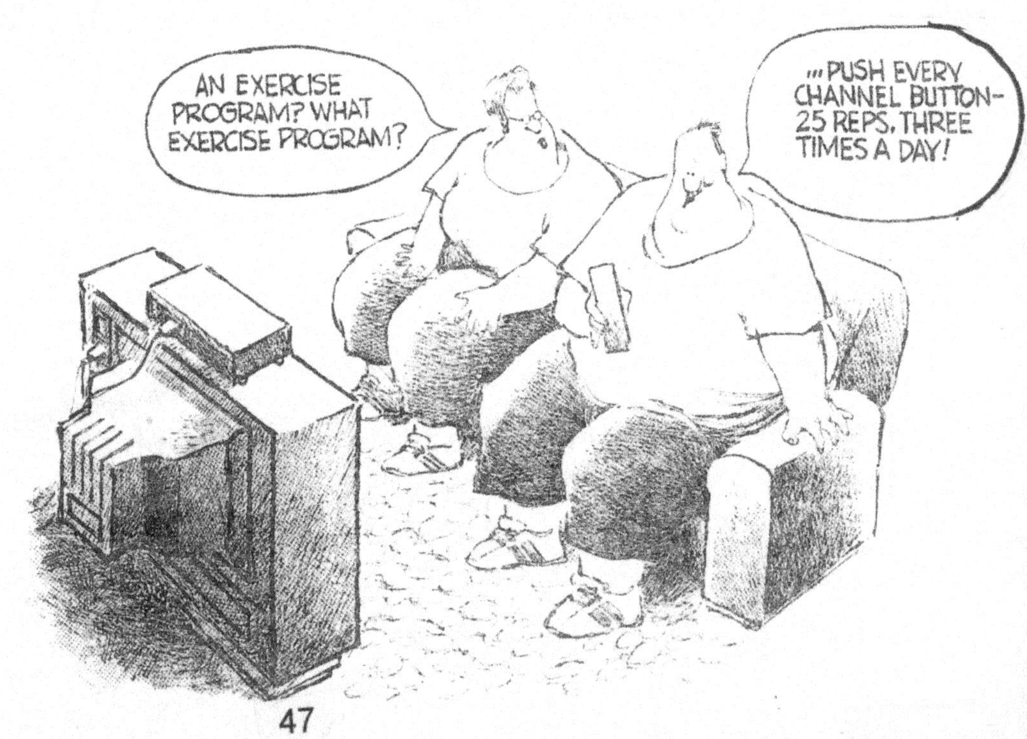

And FAT by other names is still fat.

(Painful words used to hurt and offend...)

UNSCRAMBLE THE GIVEN LETTERS TO EXPOSE "FAT" WORDS:

1. STEAB	A. FATSO	____________
2. TYATF	B. FAT ALBERT	____________
3. STUB O DARL	C. FAT SLOB	____________
4. BUTBY	D. DISGUSTING	____________
5. BRUEFBL	E. TUBS O LARD	____________
6. DRENHUT SIGHTH	F. LARD ASS	____________
7. KROPY IPG	G. SLOB	____________
8. SOATF	H. TUBBY	____________
9. BSOL	I. FATTY	____________
10. POPIH	J. FLUBBER	____________
11. AFT BOLS	K. BEAST	____________
12. DIWE-DOAL	L. HIPPO	____________
13. SOOME	M. MOOSE	____________
14. TAF TREABL	N. THUNDER THIGHS	____________
15. DARL SAS	O. PORKY PIG	____________
16. STIDGUSGIN	P. WIDE-LOAD	____________

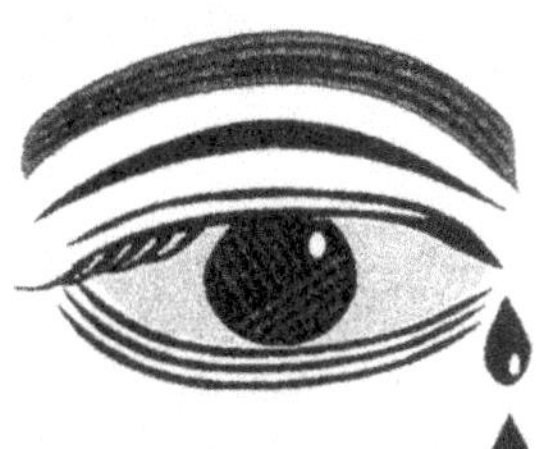

INVOLVING YOURSELF... Do you know of other names you or other overweight people have been called?

1.

2.

3.

Ann Landers counters a rude reader's remarks about obese people...

The following is a October 11, 1999 Ann Landers column:

DEAR ANN LANDERS:

"I have read several letters in your column that dealt with obesity, but I have yet to read one that addresses the fact that obesity is not a disease or a chemical addiction. With the few exceptions where obesity is caused by a glandular malfunction, it is simply caused by eating too much. Unlike smoking, doing drugs or drinking alcohol, there is nothing in food that causes a chemical addiction in the human body.

"Because it tastes good" does not qualify as a chemical addiction. Obesity is due to gluttony. There are very few signs of obesity in India. They cannot afford excesses such as overeating, so they do not get fat,

Please, Ann, let us not shed any tears for that 350-pound woman who can't wedge herself into an airplane seat. She got that way by choice. She wasn't hooked on chemicals.

If everyone ate and drank everything they wanted, the world would be full of 350-pound hippos. And let us stop putting obesity in the same category as smoking, drinking alcohol or drug abuse. Handicapped parking should not be afforded to the fat folks of the world. They are allocated for the truly handicapped, who have no control over their condition. Most fat people choose instant gratification over long-term health and appearance." - Jim in California

DEAR JIM:

"Your belligerent attitude toward overweight individuals makes me wonder what is at the root of your mean-spirited hostility. I suspect that some obese person in your childhood was mean to you.

You are wrong when you say that fat people eat too much only because it tastes good. That 350-pound woman got that way because she was trying to compensate for whatever was missing in her life by filling the emptiness with food. There is also the matter of metabolism. Some people can burn calories in their sleep, while others have trouble burning them no matter what they do. Some folks eat and drink whatever they want and don't gain an ounce. Others pay for every morsel of chocolate cake or ice cream sundae. Life deals more gently with some of us than others."

Involving yourself...

How does this article make you FEEL? ____________________________

____

____

Two big bites by
two big women
Two sets of eyes
that never meet
the waitress

Who bring them
their two big dishes:
"It's their wishes!"

(But they should NEVER eat it!)
"They're too big
and their bellies are
too fat.
They're just pigs!"

So no eyes
meet theirs.
You cannot recognize
the ridicule;
It's just a blur
If you never
look back…

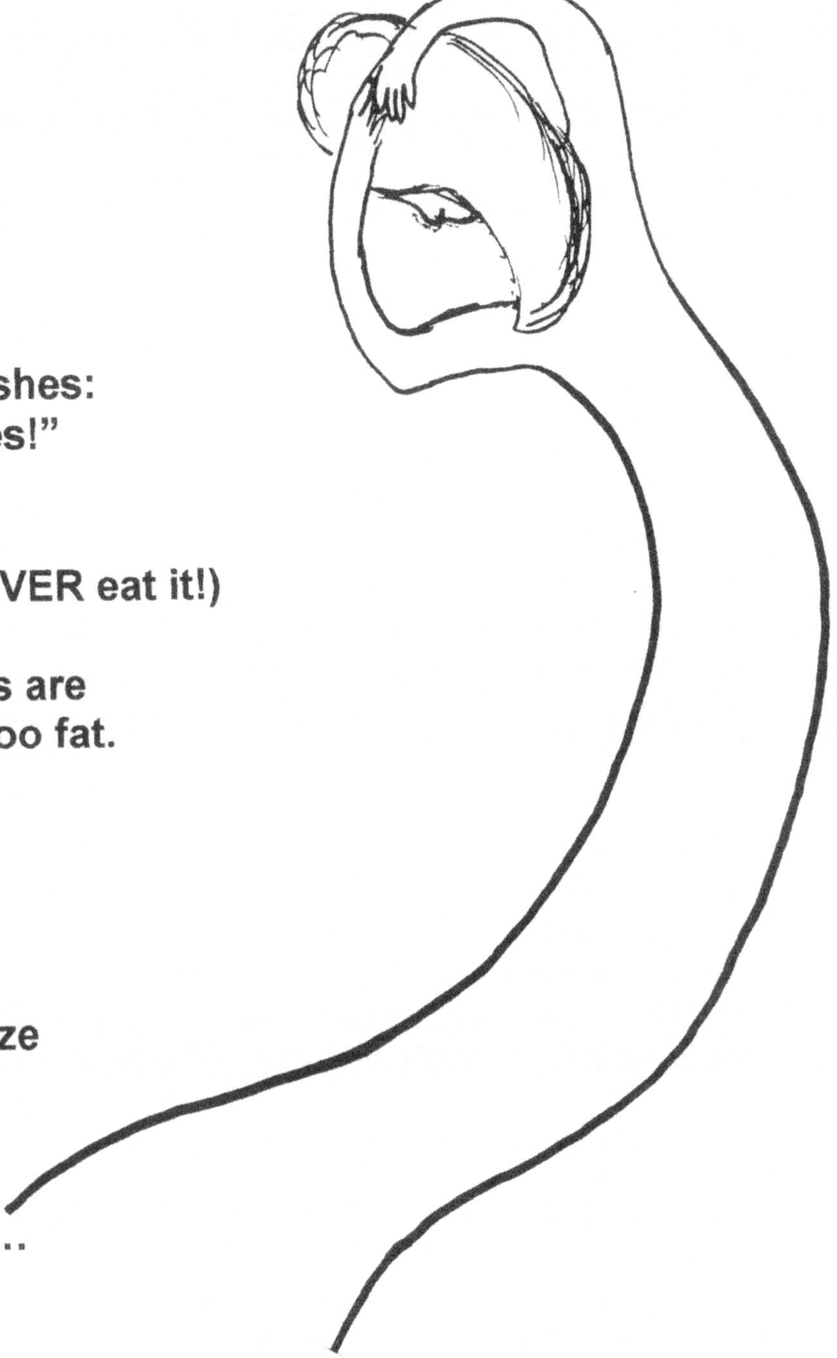

Involving yourself...

Have you ever felt self-conscious while dining in a restaurant?______

How did this make you feel? ______________________________

____

____

Many people feel it is their duty to correct an obese person's poor eating habits.

"Just stop eating out in fast food restaurants."

"Maybe you could just cut down a little."

"Why don't you start walking more?"

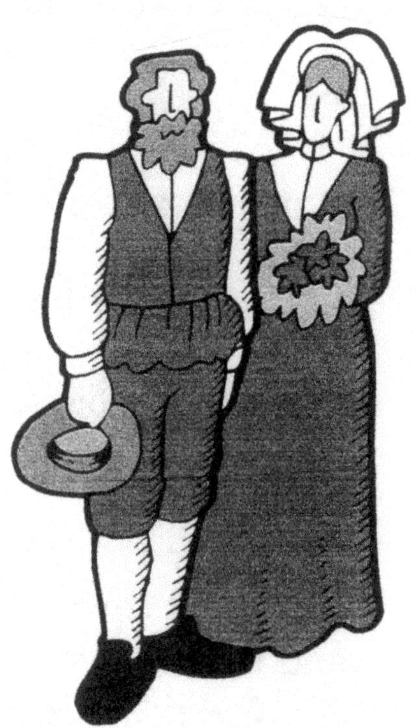

In our country, we are still influenced by our past Puritan & Protestant work ethic. The obese are often perceived as self-serving and self-indulgent, even though increasing data shows the condition is highly related to other factors. (-Esther Rothblum, University of Vermont)

HMO's and other insurance companies still want to look at morbid obesity (being 100+ pounds overweight) as a character flaw rather than a disease, even though lawyers who specialize in weight discrimination state it is discriminatory to deny beriatric surgery.

"It's like saying insurance company's will not cover cancer unless medically necessary."

Today, most insurance companies do not exclude treatment for the morbidly obese.

Involving yourself...

How does this page make you FEEL? ______________________________

____

____

____

What are the rude words used by discriminating remarkers?

MATCH a scrambled word with its correct spelling:

1. _____ gfa
2. _____ bosel
3. _____ ayg
4. _____ darter
5. _____ mulsim starretir
6. _____ knich
7. _____ hower
8. _____ tafyt
9. _____ tuls
10. _____ lawhe
11. _____ dans nomeyk
12. _____ greing

a. _____ slut
b. _____ whore
c. _____ fatty
d. _____ nigger
e. _____ sand monkey
f. _____ fag
g. _____ lesbo
h. _____ retard
i. _____ gay
j. _____ muslim = terrorist
m. _____ chink
n. _____ whale

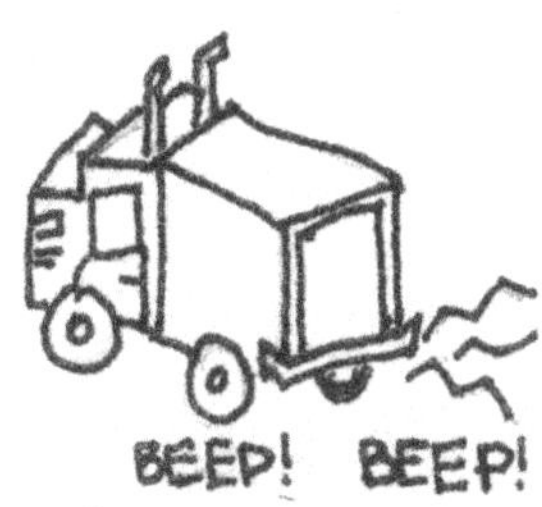

A COMMON "FAT GIRL" JOKE:

A fat woman with a beeper is mistaken for a truck backing up.

"A judgment is a continuous, high pitched, silent scream."

(- Geneen Roth, page 156)

"It hurts to listen to it. First, you try covering your ears. Then you try leaving the room. Soon you'll become frantic; you'll do anything to make the shrieking in your head go away."

Eating makes it stop.

"When I accepted the crticisms- when I tell myself I am fat- my response is to eat MORE- not less."

And sadly, your relationships sorely suffer as the personal attacks continue- until they break. Your self-hatred grows.

Judgments made fuel the flub...

Assuming you will experience future judgment assaults helps fuel compulsive eating.

Involving yourself...

How do you connect with this page? ______________________________

____

How does it make you FEEL? ______________________________

____

____

Judgments made especially by those close to you, shut down the tender parts within you...

"I felt vulnerable and started to believe I had been hit by those closest to me. I started to stop trusting them because they are not aware of my true self. I started to feel alone, like they were not on my side and that my dreams did not match with theirs.

The result was I started to shrink away from them because I didn't believe they were on my side. I felt as if I was being attacked, so I fought back- so ugly. Unfortunately, I also attacked myself and merely increased my self-loathing. The attacks themselves were my proof I had a real reason to hate myself."

Judgments crush the hope for change.

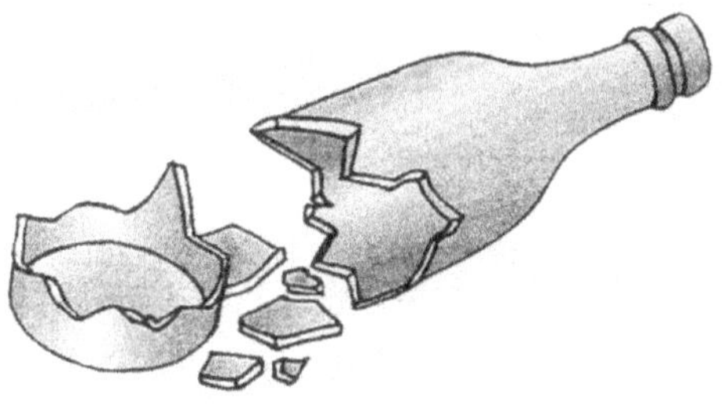

Involving yourself...

How can you identify with this page? ______________________________

____

____

____

I may be **BIG**

but my dreams are big too.

I don't hinder you by being fat.

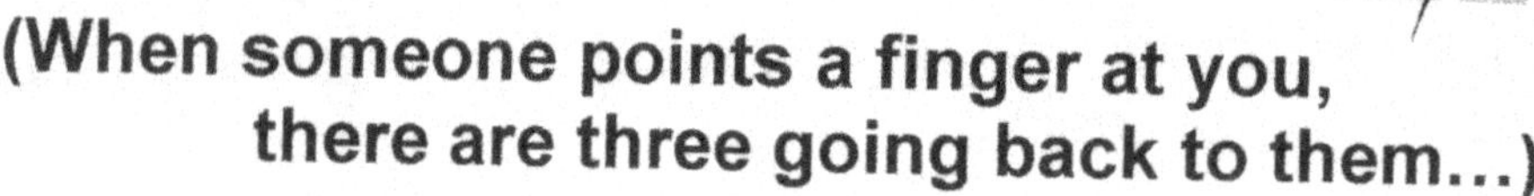

(When someone points a finger at you, there are three going back to them…)

The worst part is facing what you IMAGINE they are thinking- and judging- about you...

There are actually two TRUISMS:

1. MOST PEOPLE ARE NOT CONCERNED WITH WHAT YOU LOOK LIKE.

Most people are concerned about the way THEY look OR

They are interested in their own lives.

2. IF SOMEONE DOES THINK NEGATIVELY ABOUT YOU, THEIR JUDGMENT IS A REFLECTION OF THEM & THEIR VALUES, & LITTLE TO DO WITH YOU.

When you stop judging yourself, you'll stop judging others.

Look at those scorning you and feel bad for all the anxiety they must bear in order to keep themselves so perfect.

Involving yourself...

What do you think about this page? ______________________________

____

____

I can avoid potentially being hurt by you if I already assume you do not like me.

My fat did me well

(even though it did me, FAIL...)

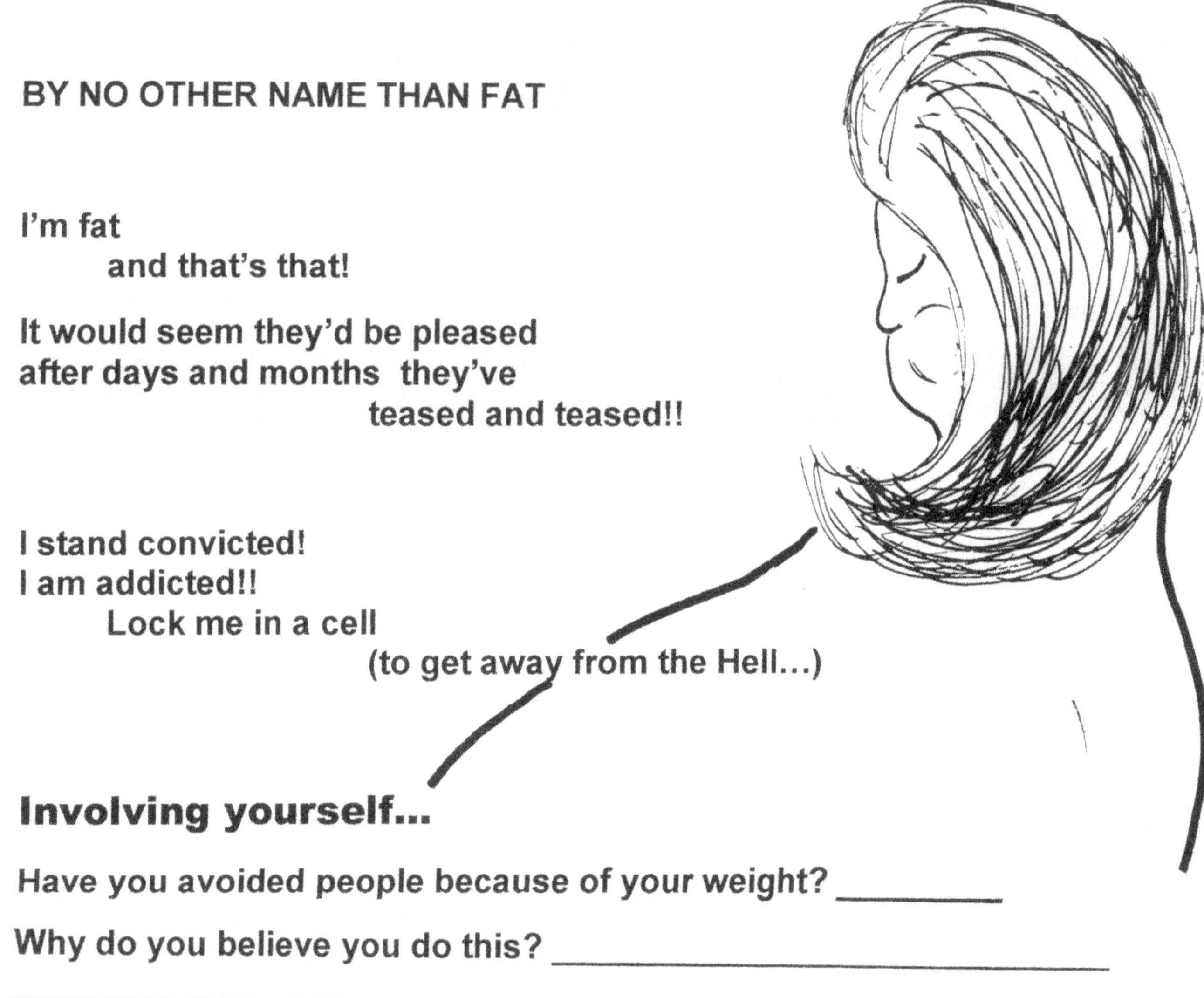

BY NO OTHER NAME THAN FAT

I'm fat
and that's that!

It would seem they'd be pleased
after days and months they've
teased and teased!!

I stand convicted!
I am addicted!!
Lock me in a cell
(to get away from the Hell...)

Involving yourself...

Have you avoided people because of your weight? ________

Why do you believe you do this? ______________________________

____

"While worrying about overeating is a cultural norm, judgments made about obese people will deny any EMPATHY for those whose eating habits resulted in being severely overweight."

- Dusty Miller, psychologist

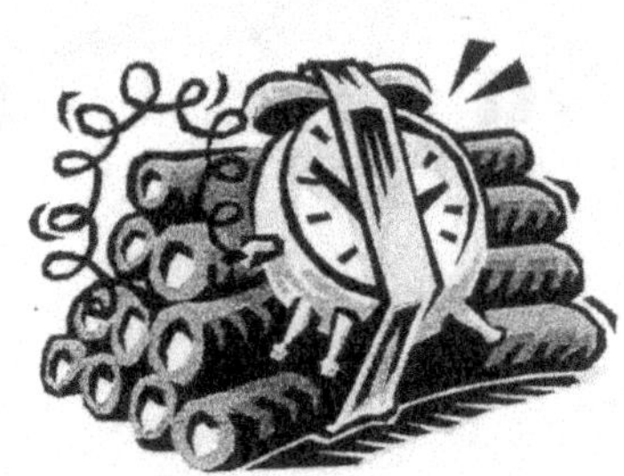

"..."... a study showed that young girls are more frightened of being fat than they are of a nuclear holocaust or their parents dying."

- Dr. Ira Sackler
- Eating Disorder Clinic at Brookdale University & Medical Center in Brooklyn, NY

Involving yourself...

How do you FEEL about these two statements? ____________________

____

____

____

____

____

____

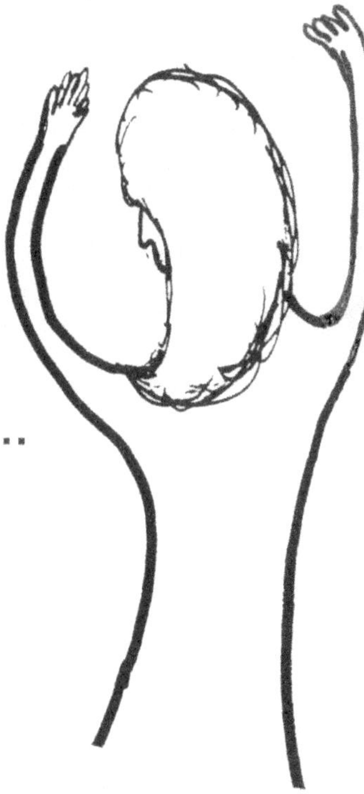

Don't turn your
nose down at me;
don't hate me:
it's not gluttony that has a hold,
But remorse and shame
that will never fold...

It's not gluttony,

it's like insanity.

Yes, GLUTTONEY is listed as one of the seven deadliest sins in the Bible. This may be a major reason the obese have endured so much scrutiny & ridicule: if the Bible says it's true, it must be!!!

A SIN???

A sin insinuates willful misconduct; an act one does because evilness has encircled your life and your soul.

OBESITY

Is not so much willful as it is closer to insanity: often deriving its power from the depths of your mind twisted and jarred apart from childhood occurrences you may have suffered through without answers.

YOU'RE NOT A SINNER
BECAUSE YOU EAT TOO MUCH.
A SIN COMMITTED AGAINST YOU MAY HAVE
STARTED IT ALL...

CHAPTER 4:

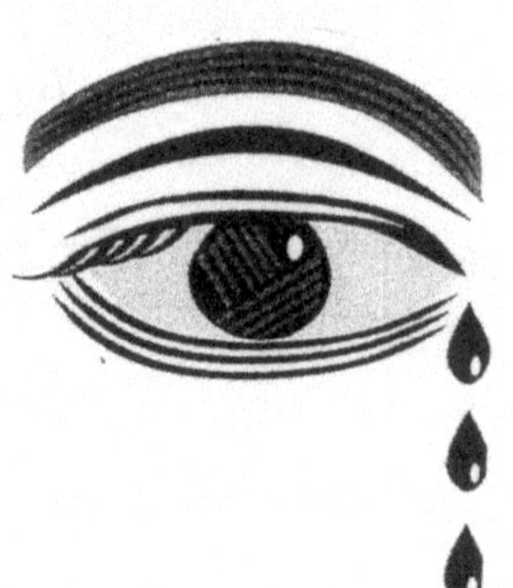

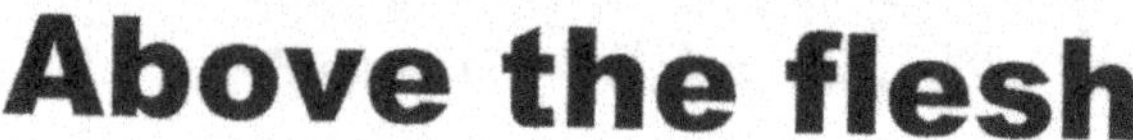

Above the flesh

On the surface:

Superficial reasons many overeaters use to explain their compulsion

I eat because food never rejects me!!

Food is always accepting; always there for you!!

We eat to celebrate;

We eat to medicate;

We eat to have a companion;

We eat to feel good.

Involving yourself...

Why do you feel you eat too much? ______________________________

For the reason you stated above, does it satisfy your need?

____

____

The Emotional Toll of being obese

"I know How You Feel"

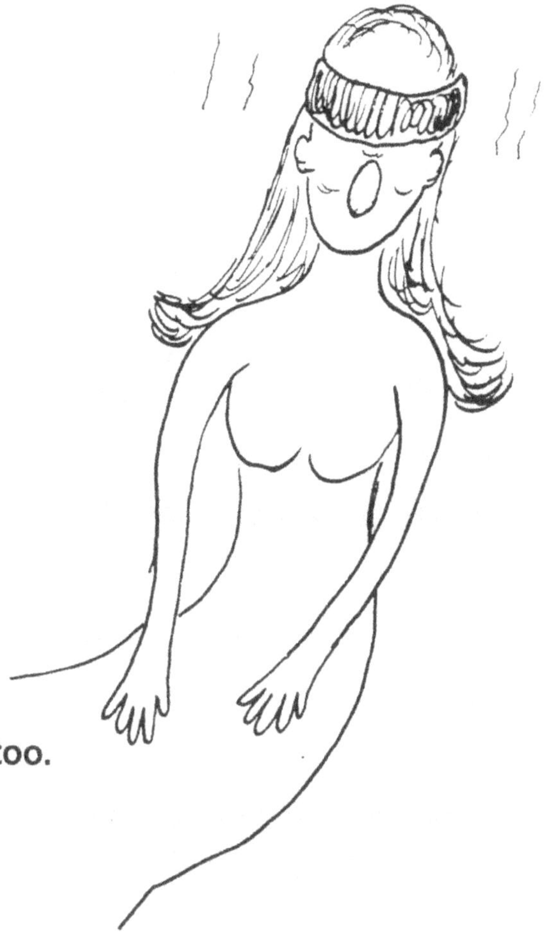

I know how you feel
sitting alone
eating quietly
your meat down to the bone.

I know how you feel
your eyes stay down
or nervously scan
to avoid knowing your frown.

I know how you feel
with your cheeks
puffing routinely in and out
to the systematic chew
you're sure to eat some dessert, too.

I can hear you cry
through the catsup on your fries;
and those refills in your cup
until every last bite is eaten up
Everybody knows you sup more when you're blue
so you will fool them too
and whistle as they replace your plate
Everyone keeps track of what you ate
Their eyes are on you.

I know how you feel
as you nervously push out the table-
just a bit-
you'll show them!!
(You'll fit there; you'll show 'em!!)

The waitress brings you more butter
and thinks you're always in need
of more feed.

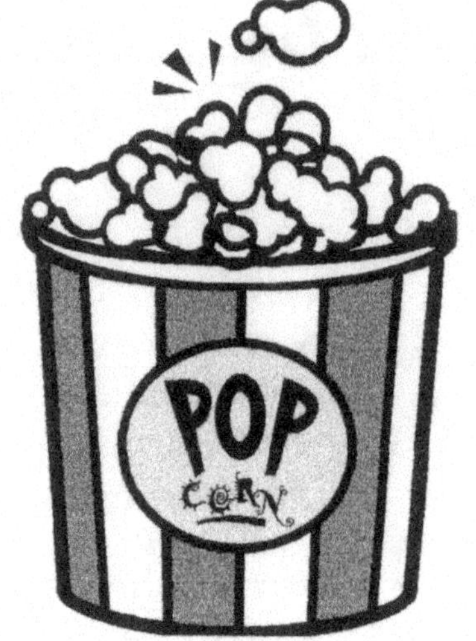

You're tired from them watching
as your cheeks puff out
like a hearthstone's billow
"For she's a jolly good fellow!"

(If they only knew how you feel...)
Your tears are real
Your laughter is hidden
under the whipped cream on your float.

FLOAT AWAY!
Is what I hear
inside the mashed potatoes hide your fears
I'll lend you an ear
BUT, I'll never watch your plate:

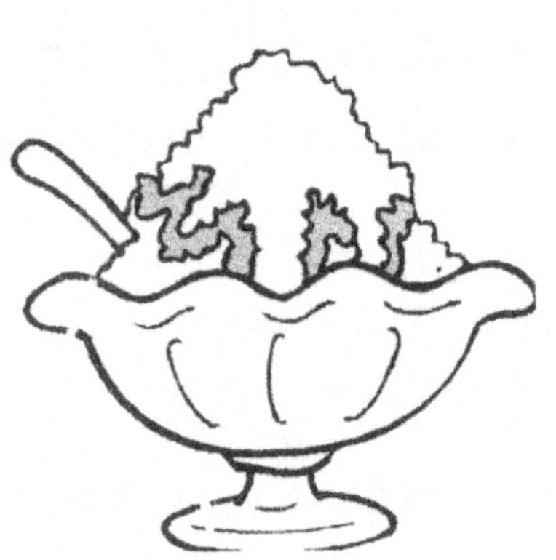

I KNOW HOW YOU FEEL...

Involving yourself...

How can you identify with this poem? ______________________________

____

____

____

____

____

____

"Here's a piece of candy for you!"

Many of us have been raised by adults showering us with goodies & treats for many special occasions or, when we suffered a boo-boo...

It's not much of a leap to see how comfort food can temporarily heal the wounds of the soul...

So when the wounds of the soul are the greatest, the need for comfort is also the greatest. Eating will soften the pain, whether physical or emotional.

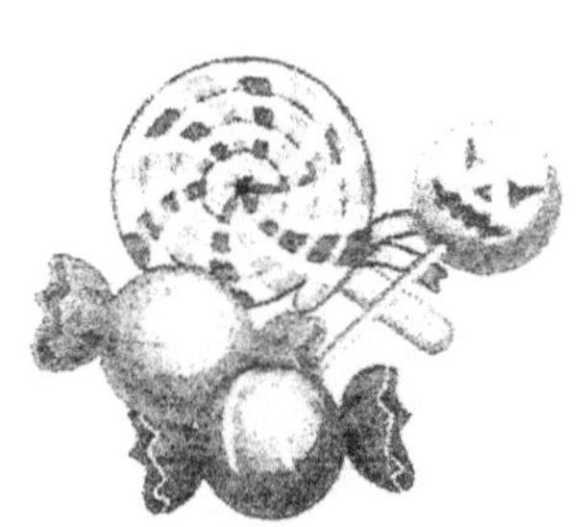

One piece becomes two;

Two pieces become three.

There's not enough for four AND me!

Ummmmmmmmm!!!

Before you know it

You've eaten more than thirty-three!!

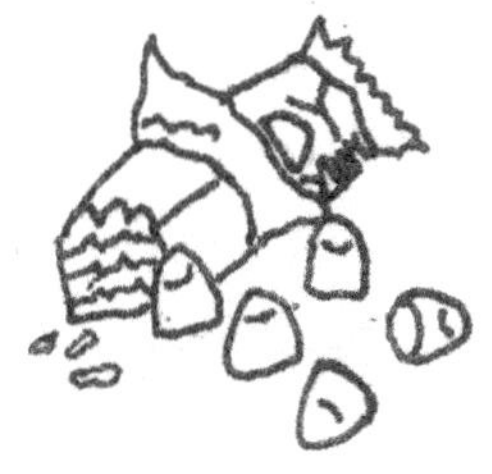

Goodies are the warm fuzzies of life! They never talk back. They never judge.

Involving yourself...

Can you see yourself in this page? If yes, in what ways?

___

___

___

To some degree, we are often ruled by our genetics.

Have you ever noticed a heavy child walking alongside a heavy mother- and possibly a brother or two? ____________________

Do you really believe this is merely a coincidence?

____

____

Then notice a tall and lean father running with his quite tall and lean son.

Again, do you really believe this is merely a coincidence?

____

____

Involving yourself...

How would you account for these differences? ____________________

____

Do you feel you are affected by your genetics in this way?

____

____

The Catch-22 of losing weight

The heavier you become, the harder it is to lose...

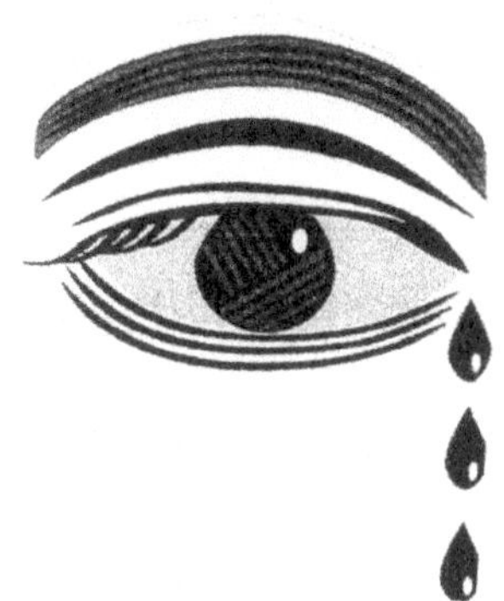

Imagine this scenario:

You weigh 250 pounds and you set out to lose weight. You develop your plan, and proudly you lose 25 pounds.

Then you really get brave and get dressed for work in an outfit you had given up hope of ever wearing again.

You go to work yearning for the praise you will receive. As you walk through the door and strut around ten of your fellow employees..... NOTHING. No one even notices and you feel crushed.

Why don't they notice? Just look at me!!

Shortly afterwards, you run to the comfort of your comfort food...

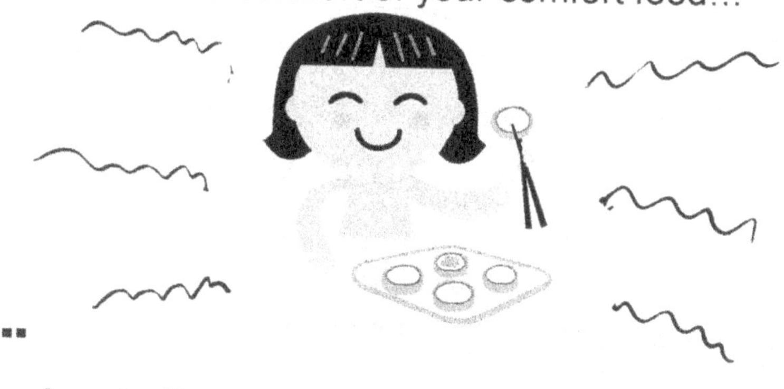

Involving yourself...

Have you ever experienced a similar experience? ____________
If so, explain below. Include your FEELINGS in your story:

____

____

____

____

Is the signal from your brain to your stomach working right???

There are huge gaps in our knowledge of weight and appetite control.

Leptin, which is a product of fat cells, literally can prevent us from overeating once we take in all the calories we need.

"You've had enough!" It hollers...

Unfortunately, it appears that some overweight people are insensitive to the effect leptin should have.

Another body-made appetite control ingredient is ghrelin, which encourages the continued intake of food.

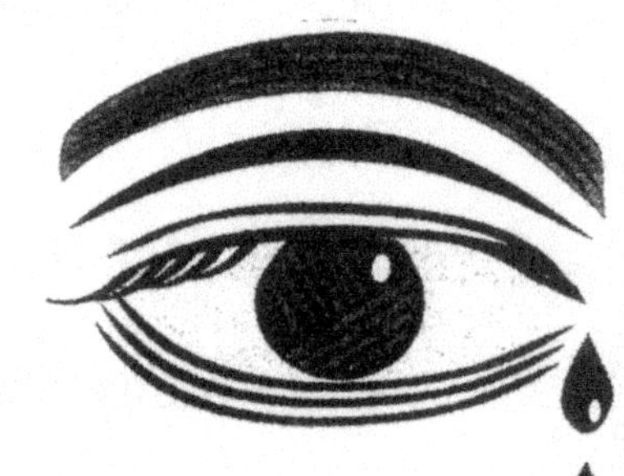

With some overweight people it is theorized that ghrelin does not shut down properly and overeaters may simply keep overeating.

However, these body chemistry quirks only work so much in explaining overeating & obesity.

Involving yourself...

Does this page pertain to you in any way? _______ If so, explain:

____

____

____

We may very well be a product of our environment...

"Monkey see- monkey do."

Mommy do- baby do."

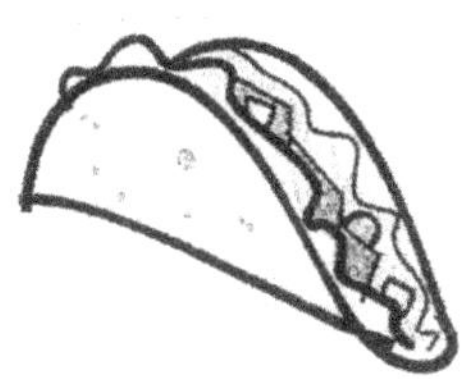

My mother made the best baked beans! The best rice pudding! Potato casserole! Potato salad!! (and dozens of other high-starch, high caloric, but oh, so good foods!)

It is so hard to give it all up...

It's very hard to walk on by when such delectable goodies cross your path.

"My mom was also obese. I can remember Friday night soda & popcorn pig outs sitting for hours in front of the TV. Every other event was about food. She too was abused and I believe she used food to avoid sex with my dad (I followed in her footsteps later in my life after a number of failed love relationships.)

Involving yourself...

Does this remind you of anytime in your past or current life? _______

If so, explain how it is difficult for you: _________________________

____

____

A legacy:

Keeping it in the family.

It's a lot easier to gain weight- and find blame- when you are raised in that "fat way."

"As much as I loved her, it seems easy to have followed in her footsteps (and my empty bowls are proof!)

Fish fries falling off the plate with French fries and a sundae topped with a shining red cherry.

Picnics held in the summer with helpings of food to go around each person three times- and leftovers to spare.

Gobble! Gobble! Turkey time for 20...

Butter cookies we gorged around the Christmas tree- just deck the halls!

Yes, FOOD!! It was my mother's pride and joy, cook so good- and her downfall... serious medical afflictions came knocking early for her, too...

Food is a fake reward for a rewardless life.

Involving yourself...

Have you used food as to escape FEELINGS in your life? _________
If so, has it worked for you? ______________________________

____

____

Eating Up Your Feelings...

There have been studies of teenage girls with eating disorders who **found that they first carried major emotional deficits- especially a failure to distinguish distressing feelings from one another and to control them- were found to be key among the factors leading to ED's.**

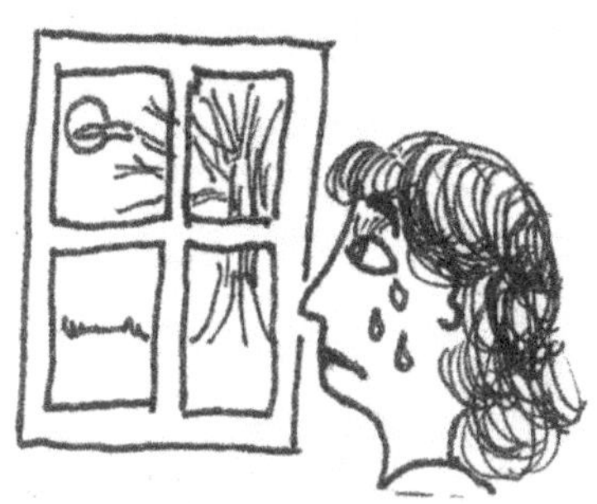

These girls were confronted with more difficult setbacks, problems and even minor annoyances with intense negative feelings that they could not sooth and less awareness of what, exactly, they were feeling.

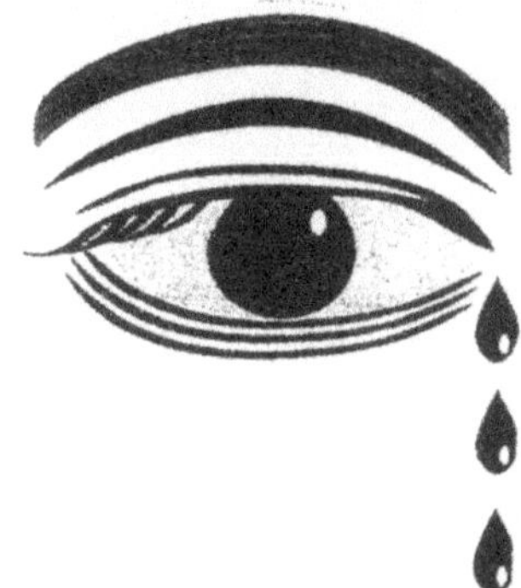

When these two emotional tendencies were coupled with being highly dissatisfied with their own bodies, the outcome was often **EATING DISORDERS.**

STRESS can cause you to gain weight.

According to researchers at University of Cinncinati's College of Medicine, SOCIAL STRESS (especially associated with relationship pressures) can often produce OVEREATING & WEIGHT GAIN- or loss.

Involving yourself...

Does this pertain to your life? ______ If so, in what ways? ______________

____

____

____

Other reasons why we overeat...

REASON:	HAVE YOU EVER ATE FOR THIS REASON?
1. **<u>The Great Reward</u>** You deserve to eat something really delectable because you were a "good girl."	________
2. **<u>The Gourmet Eater</u>** You just tingle with the taste of good food!	________
3. **<u>The Starving Children in Africa Syndrome</u>** You cannot leave food on your plate because there are children starving all over the world!	________
4. **<u>America as the Bargain Capital of the world</u>** Since the price of fast food is so cheap, why not buy it? Hey, the smorgasbord has so much to eat, so why not pile it up deep?	________
5. **<u>TV Eating</u>** Some people never watch TV without eating and never eat dinner without watching TV!	________
6. **<u>It's For Your Health!!</u>** You eat enough (and maybe too much) because you need to stay healthy and ward off starvation!	________

Still more reasons why we eat...

7. **Before-the-diet eating** ________
Since this may be your last eat-whatever-you-want dinner before your momentous diet begins, you best eat a big one! (How many last dinners will there be??)

8. **Closet Eating** ________
You only eat on the sneak, because you want to impress those around you with the strength of your willpower! (If they only knew...)

9. **Unconscious Eating** ________
You just eat out of routine- without forethought! You go to a movie and just automatically stand in line for popcorn.

10. **Boredom Eating** ________
You eat because quite frankly, you've got nothing better to do!

11. **Worry Eating** ________
When things aren't going well and you're tense and anxious, food will surely come to the rescue- at least temporarily...

12. **Guilt is the Gift That Keeps on Giving** ________
Whatever makes you feel guilty is surely helped by some special goodies! Presto! You now have less guilt! (If maybe for a while...)

"A Chinese mother told her son: Eat your food: think of all those Americans eating nothing but junk food!!"

- Geneen Roth, Breaking Free from Compulsive Eating

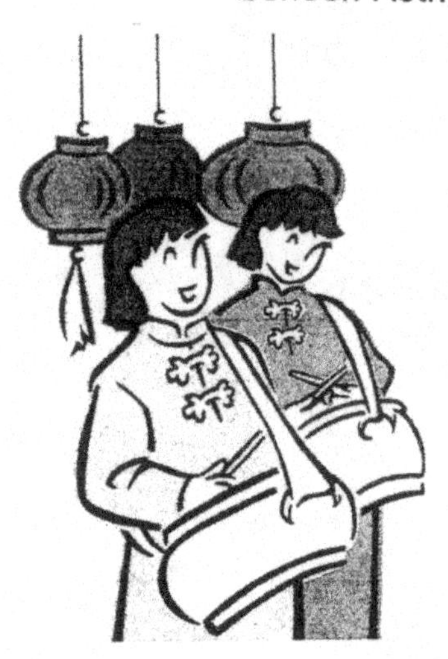

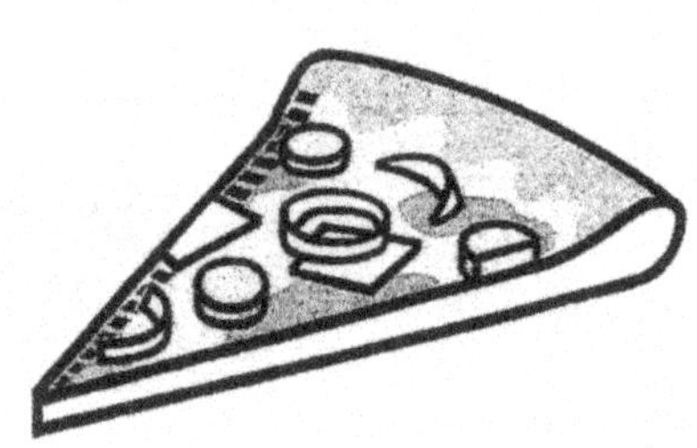

"As a kid, I was told to finish all my food- no matter what. If I wanted dessert. If I wanted to go back outside and play. Because it was good for me to eat it all up. Because mom said so. I grew up not trusting my own self for what I needed- even to eat. And my body has not forgotten…"

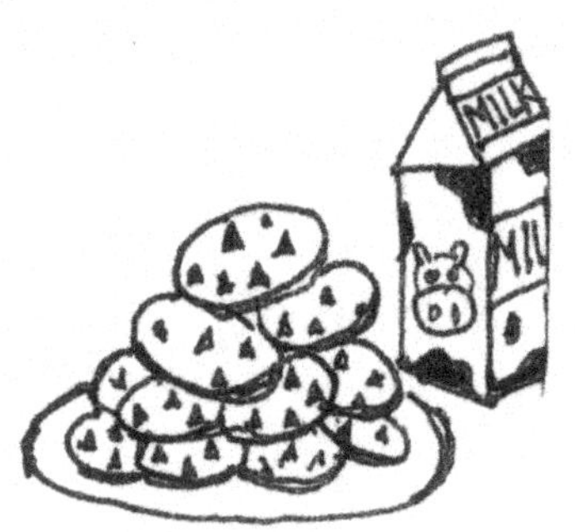

Involving yourself…

How do you relate to this page? ______________________________

____

____

____

Dessert, I presume!

OOOOOOOOOOOOOOOOOOOOOOOO!!

Look at the lovely dessert!
A picture made just
for you to see!

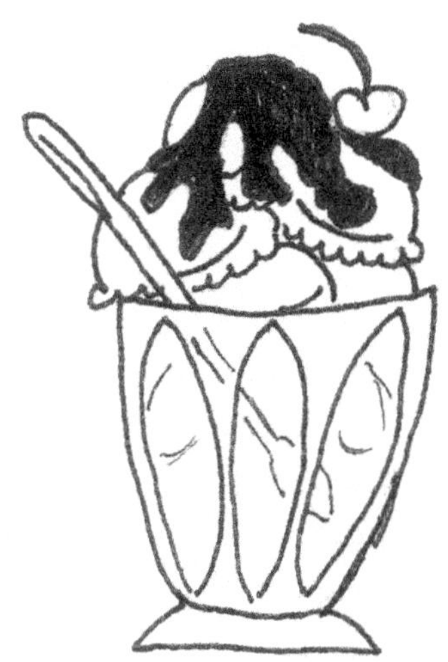

Almost good enough to eat
the sweetness just for me!
Lick, lick
so what's my pick?
Three scoops or four
After my meal
I'll surely want more??

The doorway
someday
may be hard to move through.
Maybe it's 'caus
I'm blue-
BUT...

Never mind!
I've got a dessert to disarm and blast apart!
The chocolate will slink around
my tongue,
and slick down the anals of crying moments.
And I'll gain a buzz or two.
So hap, hap, HAPPY delight!

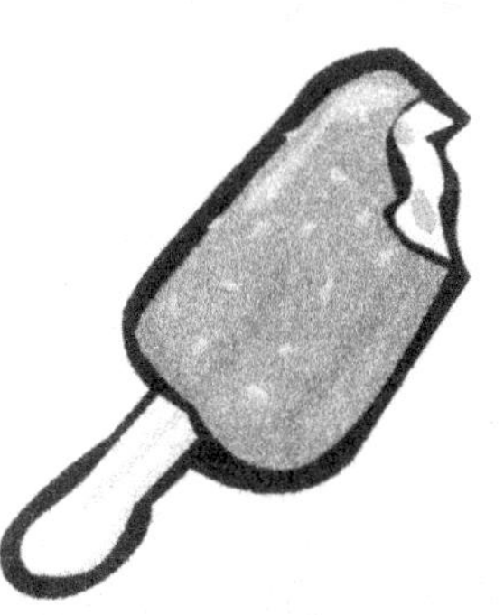

A double dipper,
a happy tripper
or a double dose of insatiable appetites
meant for one.
Just bring me dessert.

BUT, can you help me???

CHAPTER 5

Your poor health: mixing physical issues with emotional turmoil

What can go wrong physically with compulsive overeating?

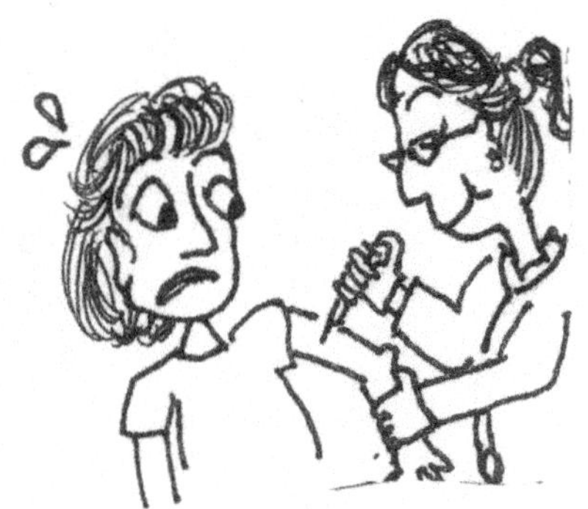

- Type 2 Diabetes (over 8% of all adults)
- High blood pressure
- Heart disease (heart attacks & stroke)
- High cholesterol
- Gallbladder problems
- Increased risk of:
  - Cancer
  - Kidney disease
  - Eye disease

Also, obesity exacerbates the affects of:

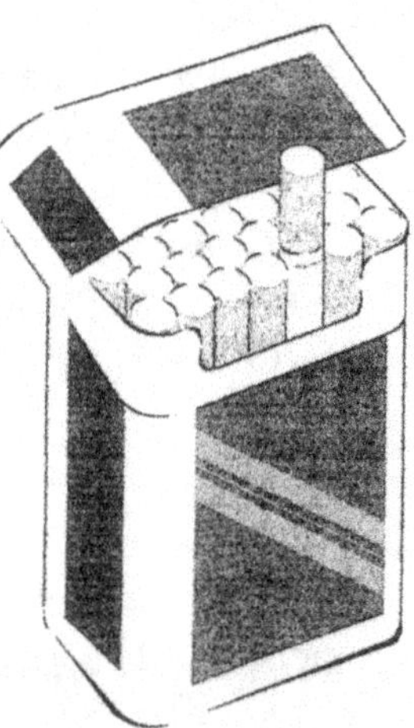

- Arthritis
- COPD
- Congestive heart failure
- Orthopedic conditions
- Depression & anxiety

Obesity is 2nd only to smoking as the greatest risk factor to ill health

Our culture is OBESOGENIC =

"tending to encourage excessive weight gain"

In otherwords, our culture actually PROMOTES weight gain.

OBESITY costs the U.S. $147 billion a year.

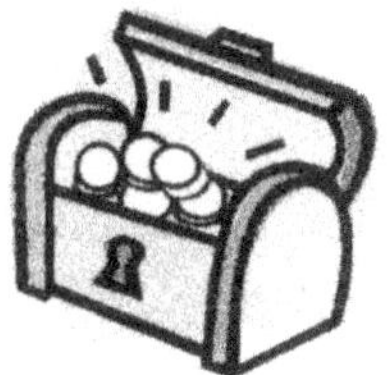

In 2015, this cost is estimated to rise to $344 billion.

Each obese person pays an average of $179,000 more for medical care in a lifetime.

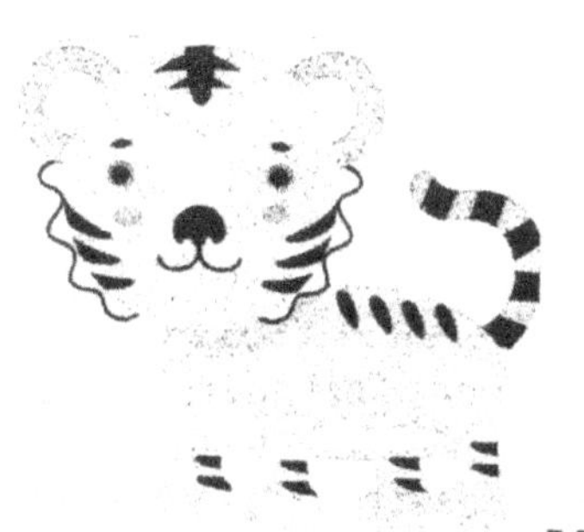

On average, the lifespan of an obese person is 10-20 years LESS than a person who maintains normal weight.

Animals eat to live,

while we too often live to eat.

Involving yourself...

How do you FEEL about this page? ______________________________

____

____

The momentum-builder for my eventual lifelong medical problems began with my diagnosis of DIABETES.

**From my onset of Type 2 diabetes in 2005,
I began to develop increasing serious medical problems.**

2006: High blood pressure; high cholesterol

2010: Heart issues (enlarged heart; irregular heart beat)

2011: ("The year of hell")

COPD (emphysema, asthma, bronchitis)
Insulin injection for my diabetes
Pneumonia
Edema
Congestive Heart Failure
Kidney compromised

2012: Orthopedic shoulder replacement
Pulmonary embolism

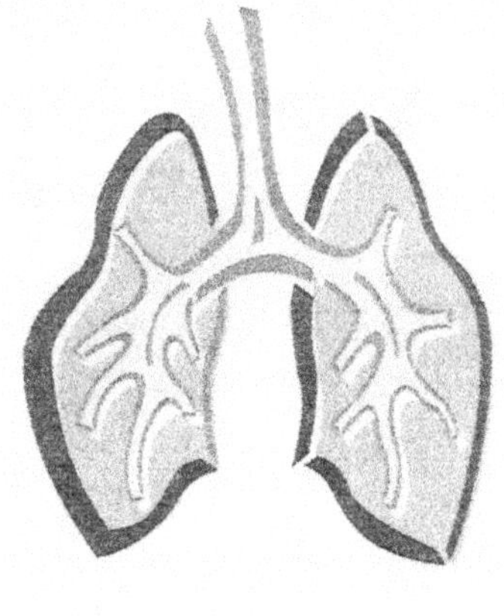

My wake-up call...

Believe it or not, I do have a positive prognosis for living more years. As I heal, I will most likely live that much longer...

Jerry Frisicaro is a psychiatric nurse serving in Buffalo, NY:

"If I see a 40 or 50 year old female client enter my office who is morbidly obese with an array of physical and mental health problems- especially depression- I could nearly be assured she was sexually abused as a child."

The spiral into further misery...

"Pretty much life just stopped around me (after my foot injury) in 2007. And all I could think about was my weight, and the more I thought about my weight, the more I ate, and then the more heavy I became, & the more hopeless I FELT, So I just continued to eat and eat out of control."

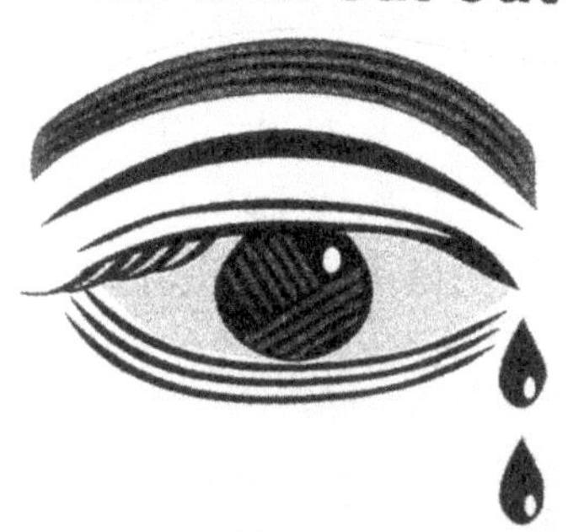

Too often the morbidly obese start to become bed-bound and then they start to lose their strength. Without use, it can take just 3 days for weight-bearing muscles to start wasting away. Lack of exercise can cause healthy muscle to lose up to 60% of their strength in just 6 weeks- and fat in the muscles begins to increase rapidly. Soon, a new round of physical problems will compound the situation, such as heart attack, stroke, kidney problems or complications from diabetes.

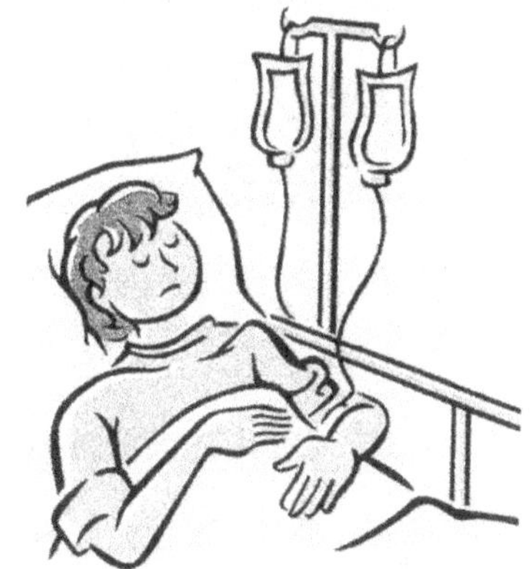

Involving yourself...

What do you FEEL about this page? ____________________

____

____

____

Why, with the associated problems of obesity, are eating disorders often only inclusive of bulimia & anorexia- without accounting for that of morbid obesity?

BULIMIA NERVOSA:

Quickly consuming large amounts of food continuing until pain. This is followed by purging, vomiting, laxatives, diuretics & enemas.

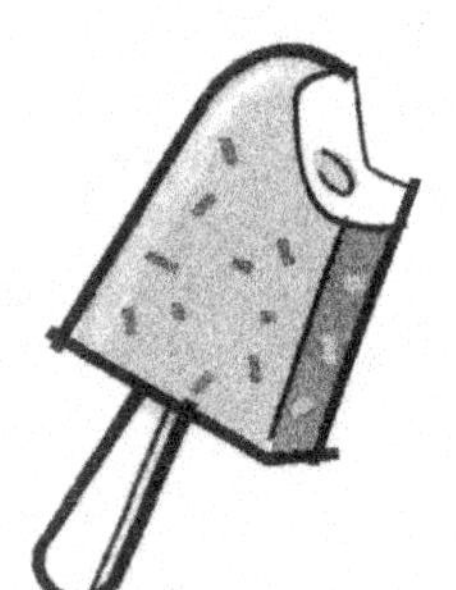

ANOREXIA:

Gradual and eventual decreasing in eatig amounts, qualities and quantities resulting in compromising health problems, especially with the heart .

Both have their roots in a culture obsessed with thinness. Under 5% of the population is affected. 55-70%+ of these sufferers were victims of child abuse.

However, 1/3 of our country is listed as CLINICALLY OBESE, many of which morbidly.

Unfortunately, most eating disorder clinics still focus its interventions on food. Chronic stress, as is derived from childhood abuse & other traumas, is an overlooked causal factor in a poor health profile.

- Lisa Ferentz, LCSW-C

YOUR BODY APPROVAL SURVEY

If you answer YES to 3 or more of these statements, you may be on your way to developing an eating disorder...

_______ 1. I am quite critical about my body.

_______ 2. I don't like to see me naked.

_______ 3. I have struggled with my weight for years.

_______ 4. When someone compliments me, I laugh it off.

_______ 5. I worry about my weight all the time.

_______ 6. I feel ashamed of my body.

_______ 7. Certain body parts of mine disgust me.

_______ 8. I can't stand to have my partner see me naked.

_______ 9. I get very uncomfortable in social situations where I believe others will watch me eat.

_______ 10. When someone I love says they love me just the way I am, I do not believe it.

_______ 11. When I see a model or other beautiful women, I feel very inadequate and think I am not enough of a woman.

_______ 12. I am always making promises to go on a diet tomorrow

It is sad even if you only answer YES to 1 of these...

A body under attack from stress =

FIBROMYAGLIA

According to Paul Donohue, M.D.,
"Fibromyalgia is believed to be an amplification by the brain of pain signals that reach it. It's like listening to a radio with the volume turned to the highest possible level at all times."

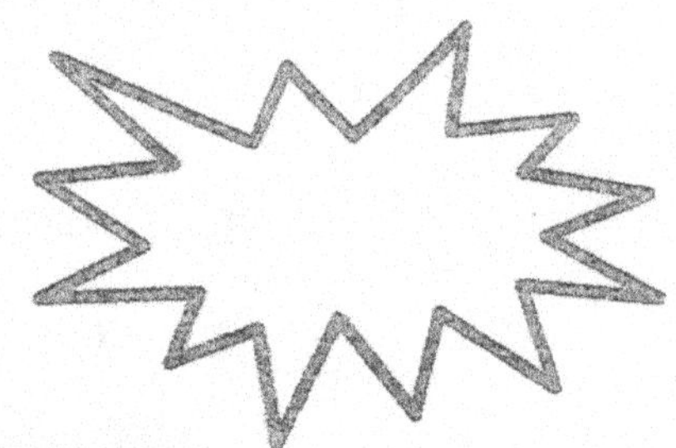

There is a growing number of researchers- with increasing evidence- that fibromyalgia could be another victim of a body under stress, often sourced from childhood abuse.

Some researchers say up to 90% of those who suffer from FIBROMYALGIA (many whom are not diagnosed yet) are actually survivors of child sexual abuse...

This increased scientific research has discovered that when a human brain is traumatized, the mind is often turned into a home for high stress & anxiety due to the unresolved abuse, which may fester and pollute for decades.

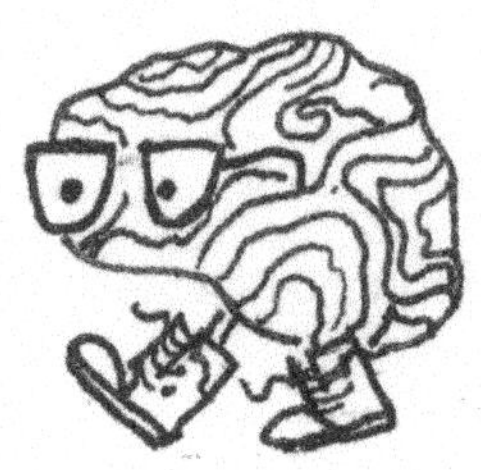

The body & brain connection has increasingly led to new understandings of what leads to some perpetual medical ills.

STRESS

does a body more harm than can be imagined.

MSNBC, 11/25/11:

Many U.S. employers are now charging more on health insurance premiums for smokers & the obese.

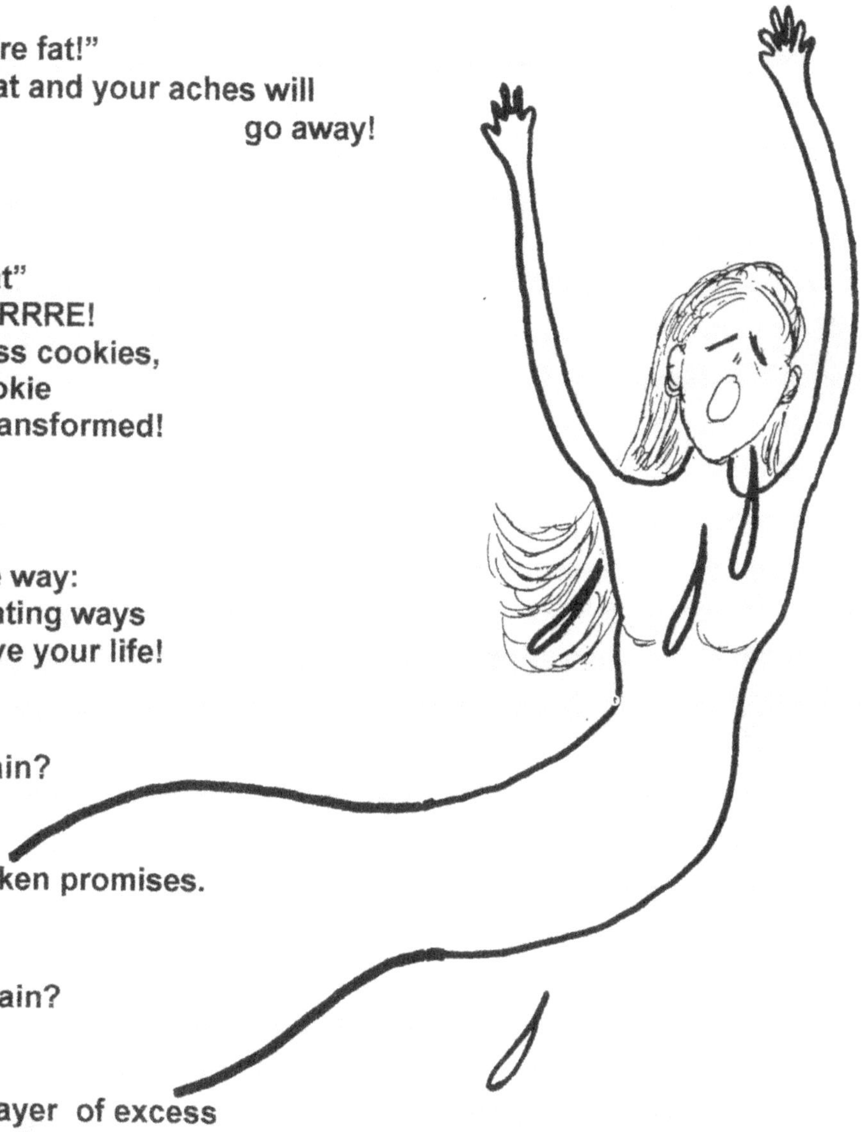

Wounded knee?
"It's 'caus you're fat!"
Don't eat all that and your aches will
go away!

"If you weren't so fat
you'd be all that"
SUUURRRRRRRRE!
All it takes is a few less cookies,
indulging in more nookie
and you'll be transformed!

Feeling tired?
The doctor knows the way:
indulge in sprinting ways
and you'll surely revive your life!

But what about the pain?
It's not just the rain
as it falls
dampening broken promises.

So, what about the pain?
"It's 'caus you're fat"
So why is it
that when layer after layer of excess
may shrink and die
my inner soul
still cries?

Can you answer me why?

I almost got what I prayed for...

"For so many years, I have succumbed to too many of the negative messages that I have allowed myself to absorb. For too many years, I have prayed to end my pain and just die in my sleep.

Unfortunately, it's never that easy. Obesity death will usually be slow and steady with increasingly more severe health issues... and chronically painful.

"You best watch out what you pray for..."

"Before I would die, I would most likely suffer from blindness, kidney problems, compromised heart and lungs- even the possibility of my toes & feet cut off from diabetic complications. It's never a "smooth" uncomplicated-die-softly-in-your-sleep affair...

But this is a slow & painful way to get 8 feet under,

SO WHY PLUNDER???

Let yourself live...

Involving yourself...

Do you feel this pertains to you, too? ______ If so, explain your story:

____

____

____

DENIAL

Is not a river in Egypt...

Even when you know it's wrong
you will eat and eat and eat;
enjoy your sweets,
indulge in your meats,
until one day- BONG!
You are knocked silly with a realization:

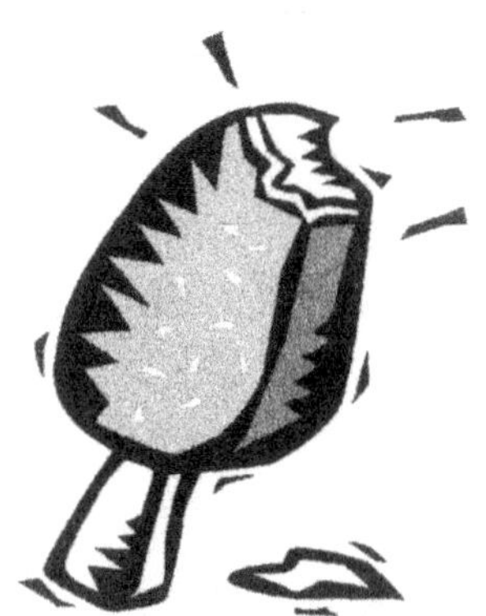

There is more than one way to kill yourself.
Your OBESITY can kill...

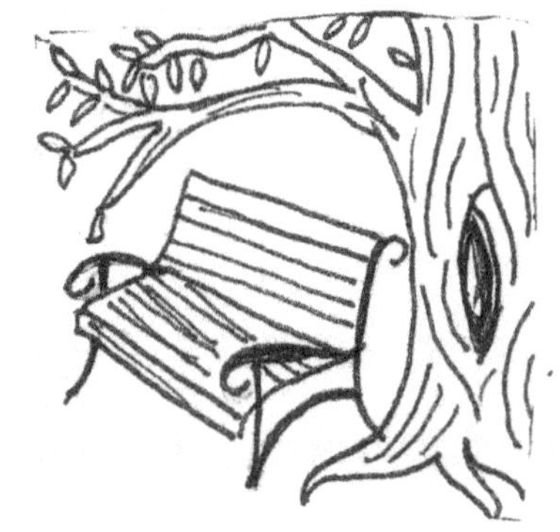

From bench to bench
 I walk the mall
 this wretched fat
 'round my legs
 keeps me lagging
and words keep nagging
 HOW DO I CHANGE THIS??

Involving yourself...

Do you trust yourself? _______ If no, why do you believe you CANNOT trust yourself? ____

____

Can you give up your hate? ______ If so, how would you do this?

____

____

How can you comfort yourself? ____________________________________

____

____

“I began to notice how much I was neglecting myself. My stress levels & my depression was increasing profusely...”

When I finally realized that the stress & anxiety were actually PREVENTING my upward climb towards recovery, I also discovered that my MENTAL HEALTH, which is connected to my PHYSICAL HEALTH, was then preventing any attempt at weight loss!”

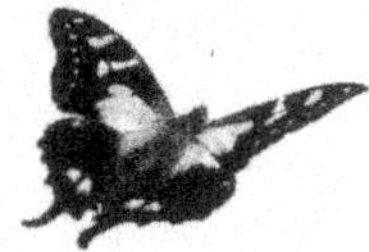

Therefore, I soon accepted the fact that unless I addressed my MENTAL HEALTH (which centered on any recovery from the devastation I still harbored from my early child sexual abuse.)

Without this healing process, I will continue to spin in the same circle over & over, while I continue to experience uncontrollable eating.

It IS time to get going & start healing!

Involving yourself...

Are you ready to get healing??_______ Are you prepared? _______
If so, are you ready to start the long and even treacherous journey to recovery by opening your mind and working to expose- and then erase your demons? _______ When will you start? _________

Chapter 5

THE MOST DIRECT & HORRIFIC CAUSE OF OBESITY?

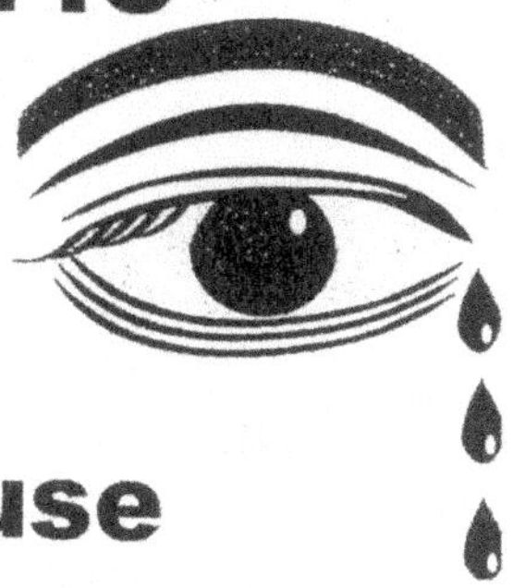

=

Being a survivor of child abuse (sexual, physical & emotional), neglect & abandonment

At least 65% of those individuals with morbid obesity have such a history in their childhoods.

You may ask WHY this is true?

When children experience child abuse, most are literally brainwashed with negative messages about themselves. These messages include those which scream through their brains: "It is your fault! You deserved this happening because you are bad!"

Most morbidly obese individuals do not lack willpower & resolve: they lack self-worth, esteem and often, HOPE…

1 out of 4 girls & 1 out of 5 boys have been sexually abused. 1 out of 3 children will experience some form of abuse, neglect and/or abandonment. From these numbers, approximately 70% will experience some form of social, economic or physical affliction.

These numbers account for a great deal of hopelessness…

The Child Sexual Abuse & Obesity Connection

According to national statistics, 55-70% of the morbidly obese have experienced one or more incidents of child abuse, neglect and/or abandonment as children.

- North American Association for Study of Obesity; The Post Standard, Syracuse, NY 2011

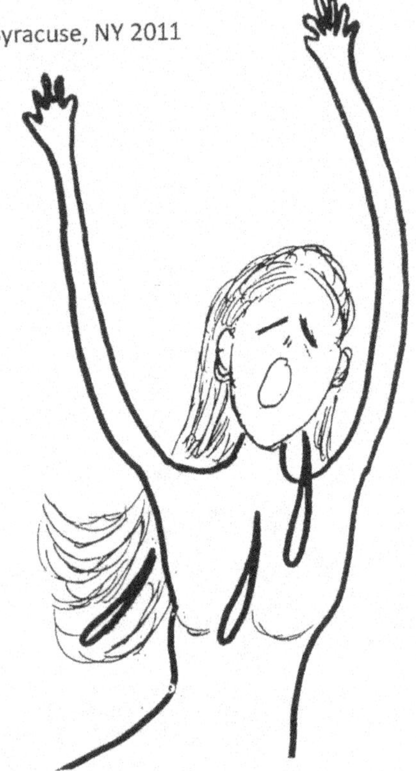

There are tears in the heart that never reach the eyes.

Notable celebrities who have been abused & have struggled with obesity:
OPRAH WINFREY, RICKI LAKE, ROSANNE BARR

(By some trauma experts, only 25% of actual survivors have admitted it to others.)

Involving Yourself . . .

Do your tears reach your eyes?____

____

The biology of your cravings . . .

When cravings strike, they can consume every thought in your mind until they are satisfied. Just thinking of that special food can launch the body into a feeding frenzy of pre-digestive action.

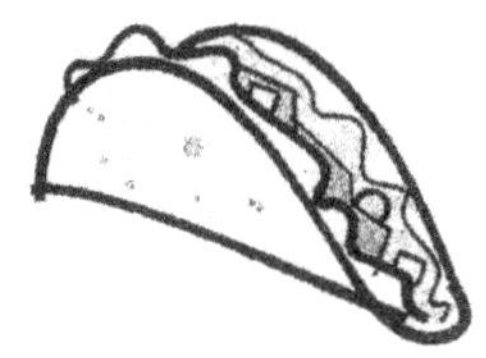

Your heart races, your salivary glands start flowing and your stomach secretes acid in a "ready-set-go" fashion. Insulin is released, causing a drop in blood sugar levels that actually leads to more hunger.

When you are under stress, or when you have led a stressful life due to childhood traumas, the act of digesting food turns off that part of the nervous system that makes you tense, so it can act as a relaxant. Then there is a release of the calming chemical, serotonin.

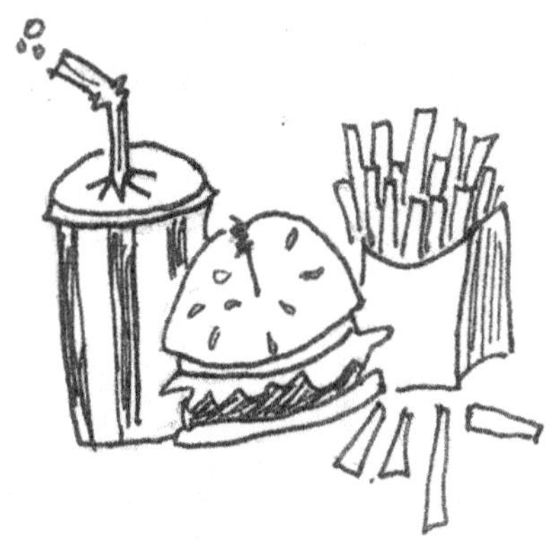

Unfortunately, when you are a survivor of childhood abuse, your brain may have been most likely altered to produce LESS feel good chemicals.

Your brain may have lost the ability to satisfy the craving. With no "I feel better now" messages coming from the brain, you keep EATING,

And EATING,

And EATING...

Your favorite goodies may just boost the potent brain chemical called serotonin, our "feel good brain chemical."

When your serotonin levels are boosted, it screams out:

GIVE ME MORE!!

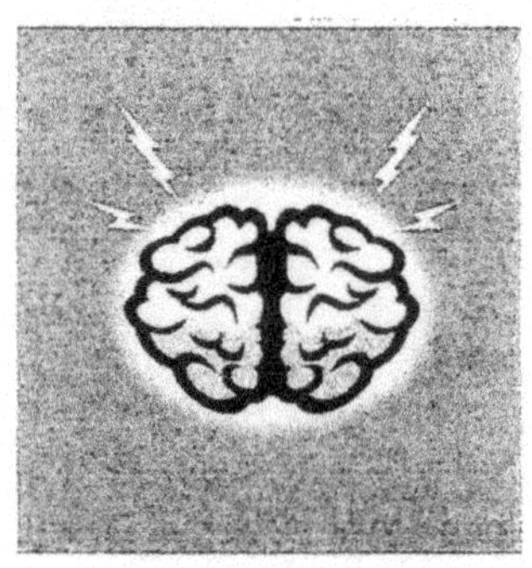

This may be especially true of people who have experienced some form of trauma, especially childhood abuse, neglect and/or abandonment. Under such anxiety stemming from these horrors, many develop an over-reliance on other means of self-calming and soothing.

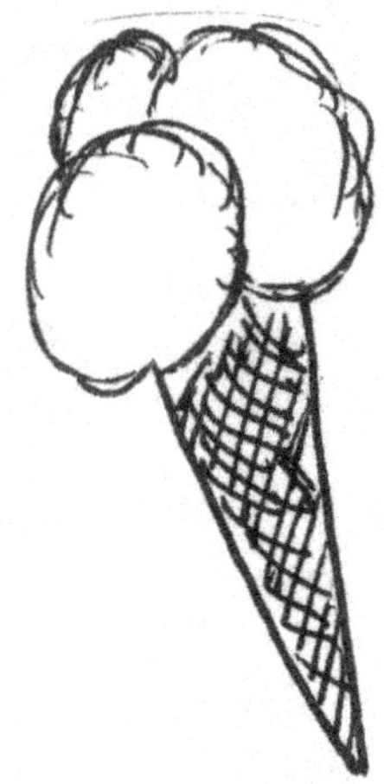

Unfortunately, this manner of feeling better by relying on extra "doses" of serotonin is also believed to be the root of many addictions, which can include compulsive overeating.

Involving yourself...

Do you believe this pertains to you? ______________________________

If you do, how do you respond when you feel obsessed? __________

____

____

____

Cravings can be as powerful as those of a drug addict or alcoholic...

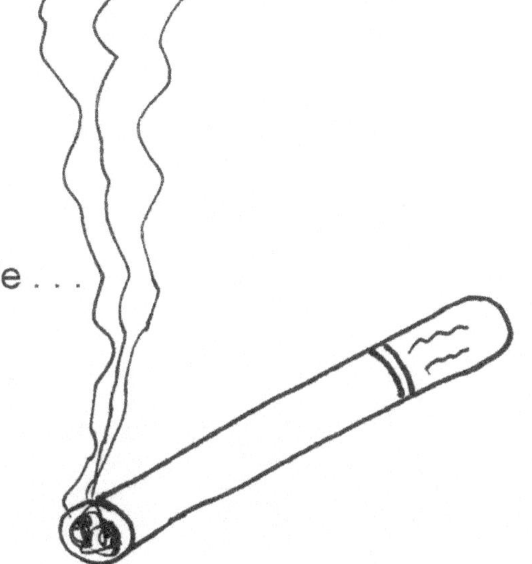

As a young woman, I turned to mind-altering substances to get me through the night and to forsake my pain.

Alcohol worked for a while . . .

Sex tried its best but failed along with those I wouldn't- or couldn't- trust.

I puffed and puffed those cigarettes day and night, with food or without.

Food was the worst craving I ever experienced.

Involving yourself . . .

How can you relate to this page? ______________________________

____

Have you tried other ways to calm down and feel good? __________

Explain: ______________________________________

____

Did these substances work at first, but not as time went on? ______

Did the other substances affect you negatively? __________

Compulsive Overeating fulfills the definition for an addiction.

Your overeating becomes #1 in your life.

CHARACTERISTIC:	DOES THIS FIT YOU?
1. You can't seem to quit thinking about food.	____________
2. You cannot seem to quit.	____________
3. You engage in "sneaky eating".	____________
4. You deny the amount and frequency of your habit.	____________
5. It often dominates your thinking.	____________
6. You plan your day around your eating.	____________
7. It is your #1 relationship.	____________

If you answered YES to two or more, you may very well have an addiction to your overeating.

The greatest challenge to quitting is that you cannot completely quit eating . . .

Involving yourself . . .

Do you ever feel your eating is an addiction? ____________

If so, explain here: ____

____

The self medication cycle

The following diagram illustrates how a survivor of trauma can too easily become an abuser of substances & alcohol.

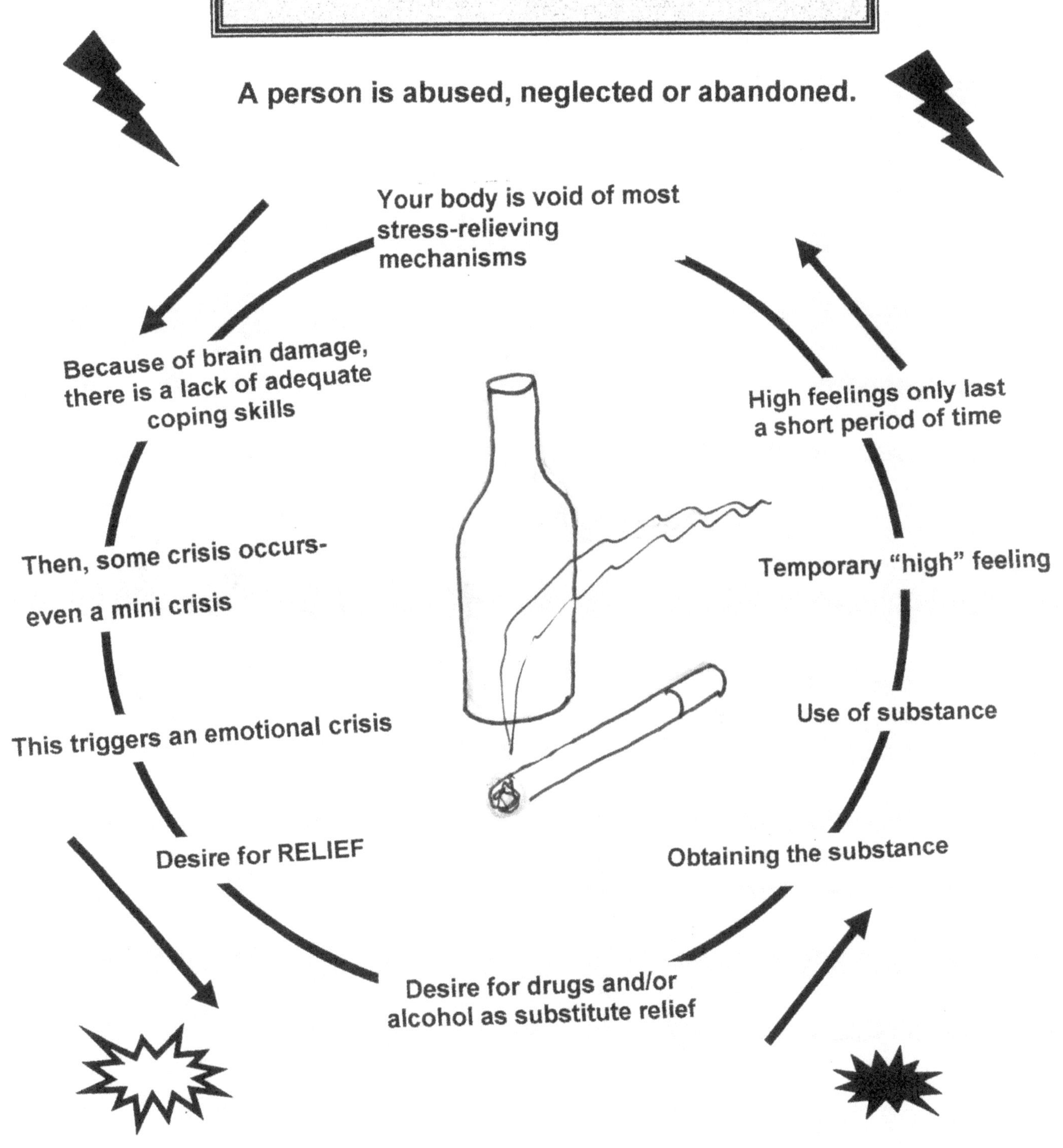

My heart
is buried deep,
(so well hidden)
that I can keep
you far away from me.

Maybe this is why
I grew
this fat around my soul
because I knew
it could keep me from trusting you.

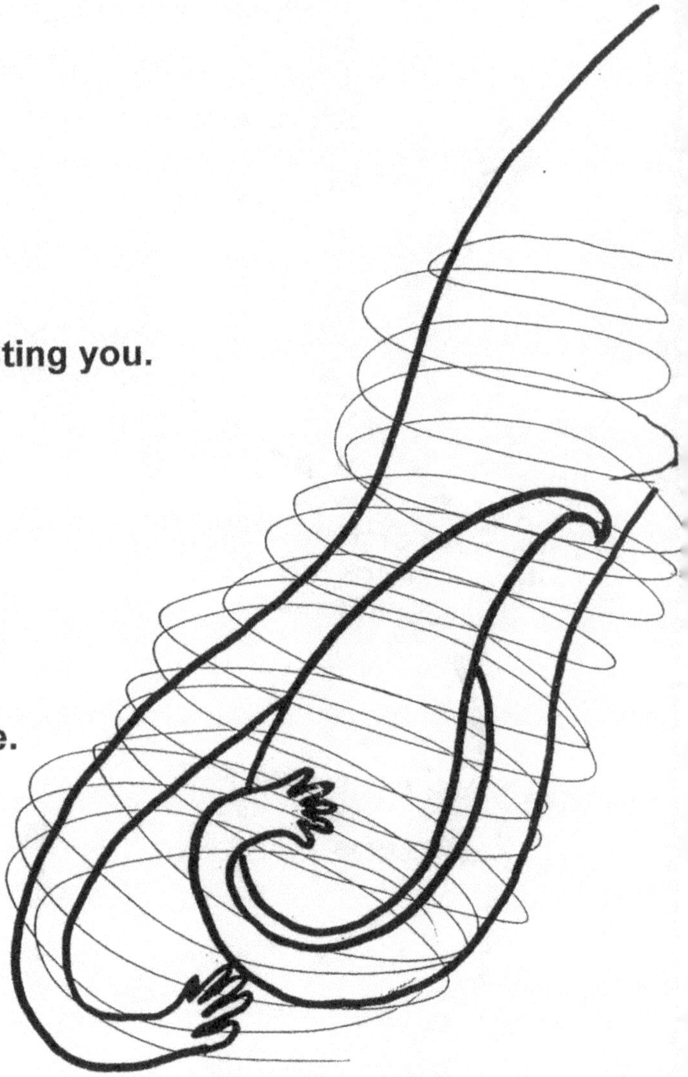

I can sit here
and eat for two
(but only one fork!)
and maybe I can fool
you from seeing I sit alone.

Why can't I stop?
Why can't I push the plate
away
even after I'm full?
It's not from waste
it's not that it all tastes
so good
because actually you see I feel so bad.

Why can't I stop?
Why can't I push the cookies
on that plate
(or some candy I wish I'd hate!)
Sure I'm full
Yes,
Why can't I stop?

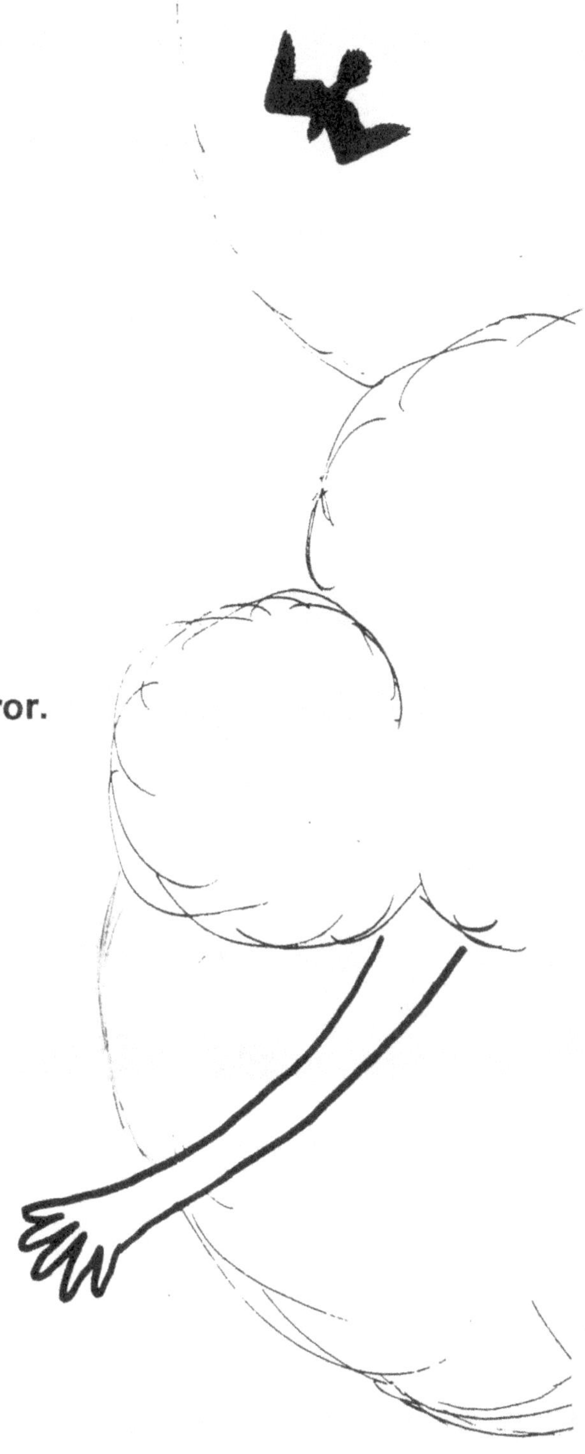

Why can't I stop
Do you think I like my hand
trying to cover
up my gut
or avoid getting involved
Do notice how I scoot by
hurriedly
whenever I pass by a mirror.

So why won't I stop
a nagging question
EVERY day
as it plays down
on my self-esteem
(I can only scream)
Help me!
Because I can't seem to stop
But,
STOP
(don't come too close...)

Involving yourself . . .

What parts of this poem can you identify with? ____________________

____

____

____

____

In my own clinical psychologist work, I find that women who have developed patterns of seriously self harmful behaviors (such as eating disorders) are unlikely to do such things to themselves without an underlying history of abuse or neglect.

- Dusty Miller, Clinical psychologist and writer of *Women Who Hurt Themselves,* 1994

" I did not remember my abuse incident for 25 years after it occurred, yet I discovered how much my life- with all its problems and defeats- had been motivated by the subconscious workings of this abuse..."

Abused...

The Touch that Kills

SHHHHH!!
I can't tell Mommy.
If I did,
she'd ask me why,
and I've been so bad I just want to die...

This man
gave me the touch that kills,
and I cannot forget,
with all the booze and many pills.

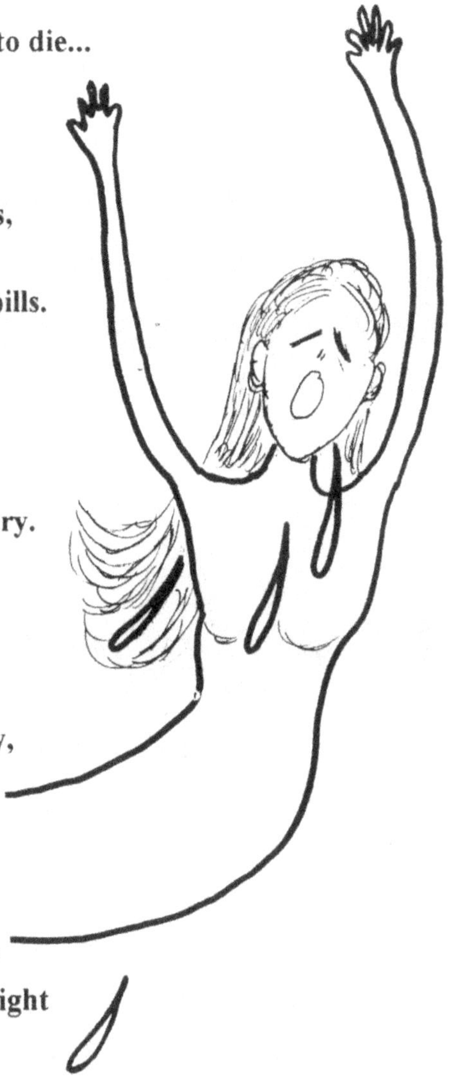

SHHHHH!!
I can't tell my mommy:
the shame's so deep I could cry.
He said I had it coming,
so now I live a lie...

She'd tell me I was naughty,
or I was bad.
I can't make her angry;
I can't make her mad.

Sh, so I can't tell Mommy
'cause she may think I'm all right
still-
But it's hard to believe
with the touch that kills...

WHY?
THE SEXUALLY ABUSED JUST ASK WHY THEY FEEL LIKE THEY DO.

What are the underlying results of sexual abuse? Refer to specific lines in the poem, *The Touch That Kills.* Then, MATCH it with its often hidden meaning.

(1) *"I can't tell Mommy!"* ______

(2) *"...I've been so bad I just want to die..."* ______

(3) *"and I cannot forget, with all the booze and many pills."* ______

(4) *"She'd tell me I was naughty, or I was bad."* ______

(5) *"But it's hard to believe,"* ______

(6) *"with the touch that kills."* ______

a. Victims too often experience low self-esteem and insecurities.

b. Sexual abuse victims often try to hide their pain by the use of addictive substances.

c. Children of sexual abuse often do not tell their parents, since they fear being punished.

d. Childhoods, innocence, and dreams often die along with the spirit of the abused.

e. Abusers often "teach" victims they deserve the abuse. The child may actually fear parental punishment!

f. Abuse victims often feel used up and no good.

Child abuse weakens the foundation of a survivor's life...

Childhood is the time when personality & mental development is formed. When a child is abused, their sense of trust & faith in the world is too often shattered. When emotional development is stunted, so might one's life- sometimes forever. Too often, survivors go through life weakened, negatively altered & scarred.

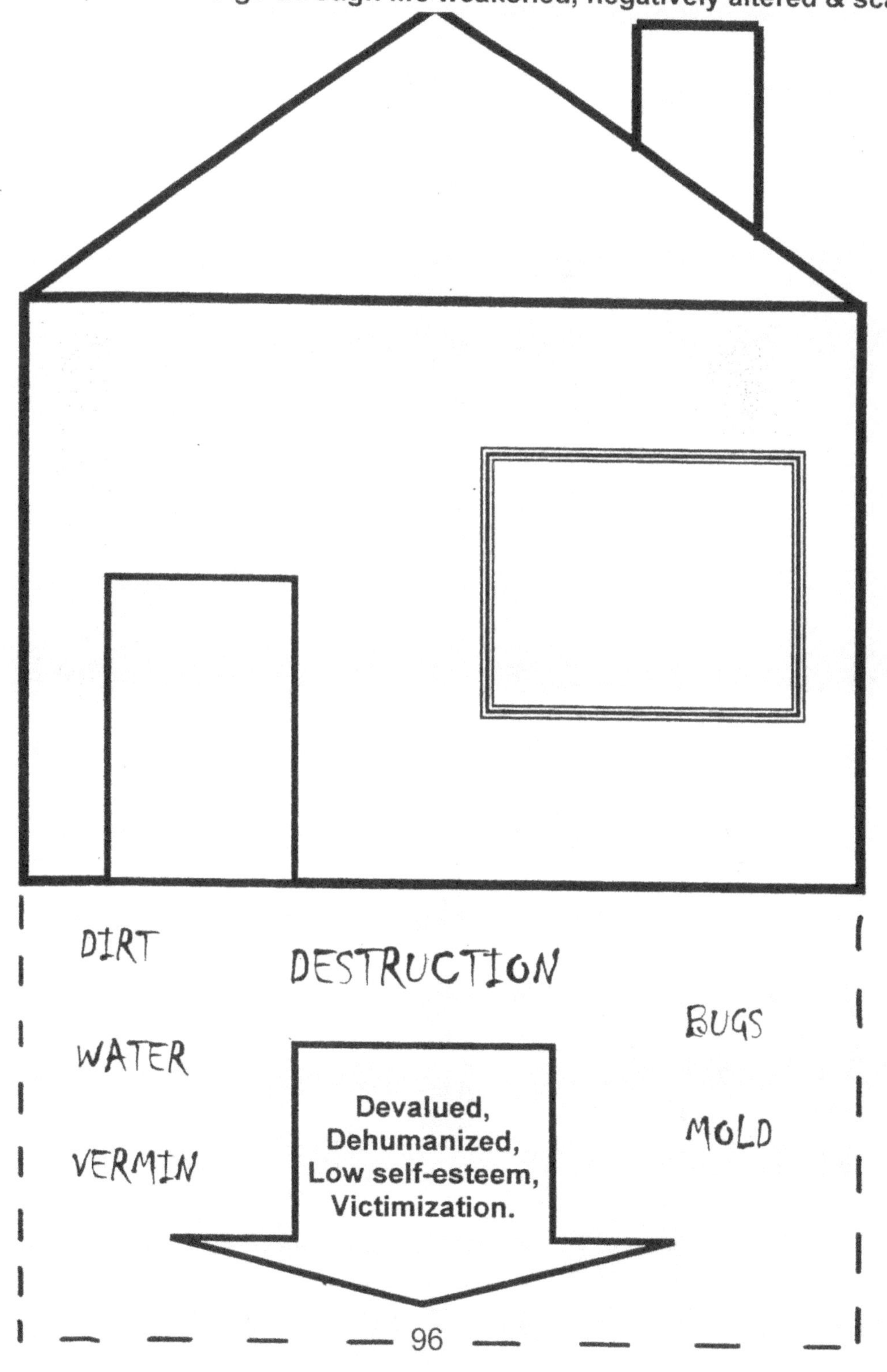

"I happily went to my daughter's first kindergarten open house. All the children had drawn a drawing of themselves. Most were brightly colored with smiling, happy scenes. THEN, I came upon my daughters:

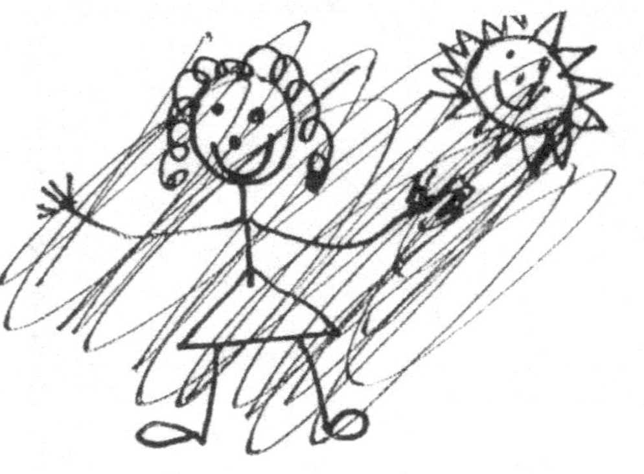

SELF-PORTRAIT OF A 5 YR OLD SEXUAL ABUSE SURVIVOR

"When a therapist asked a 7 year old boy about how his sexual abuse experience felt, He would not answer for a long time. He stopped drawing a picture of his family with

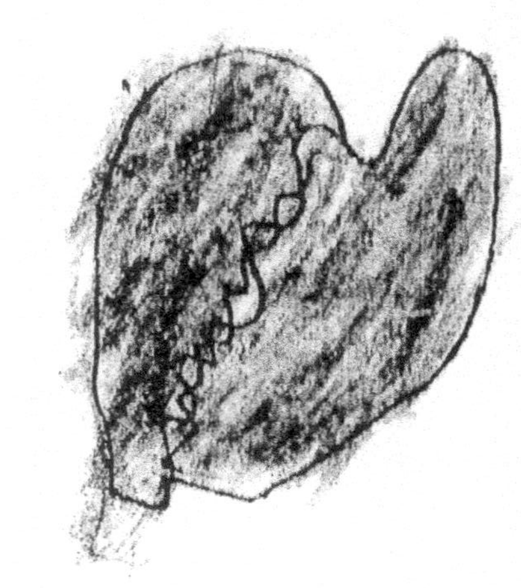

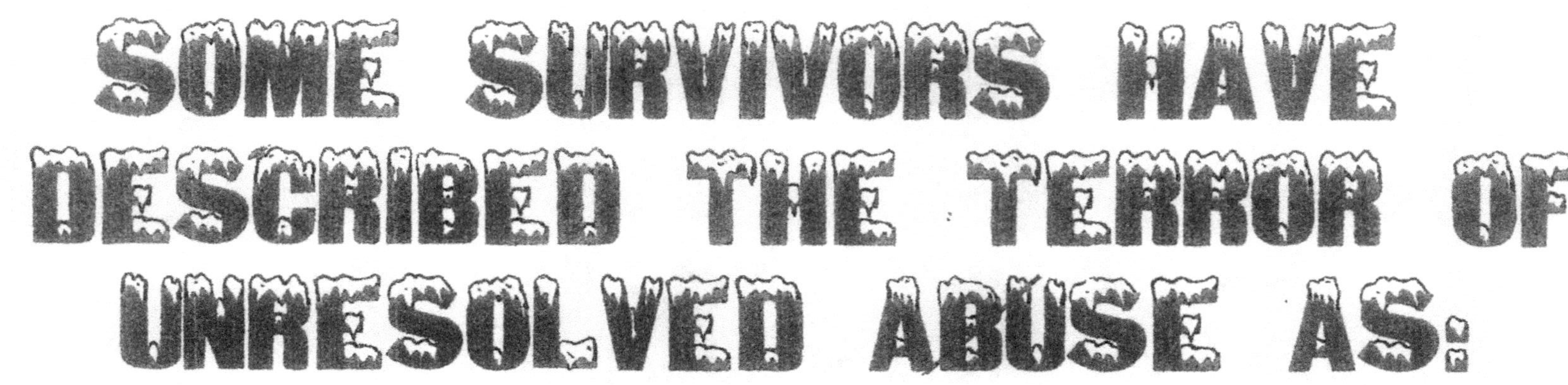

"Silent screaming with
your mouth wide open..."

"If there is anything
new to jar me, I will explode!"

"...something
so bad I'll never put
the pieces back together again."

"...fear of crying
that will never end"

"My depression
Is like frozen rage"

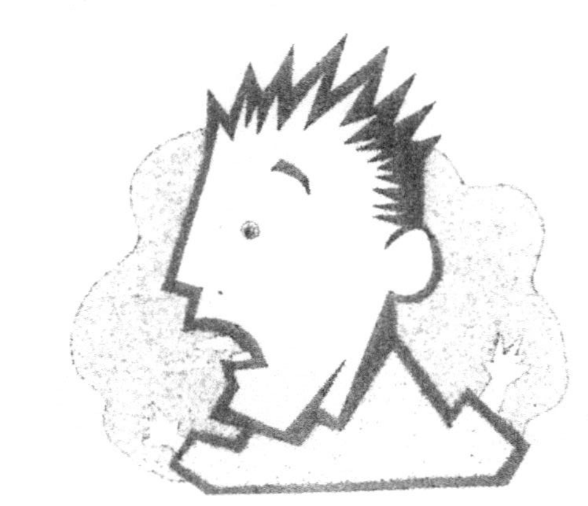

"Fear of what will happen
in the dark afterwards..."

"Fear of what tomorrow
will bring..."

COMMON REACTIONS TO TRAUMA

- Fear & anxiety
- Re-experiencing of the trauma
- Increased arousal
- Negative world view
- Feeling angry & irritable
- Blaming themselves for how they survived
- Negative self-image
- Difficult to trust others
- Feelings of going "crazy" or "losing it"
- Feeling that the world is a dangerous place

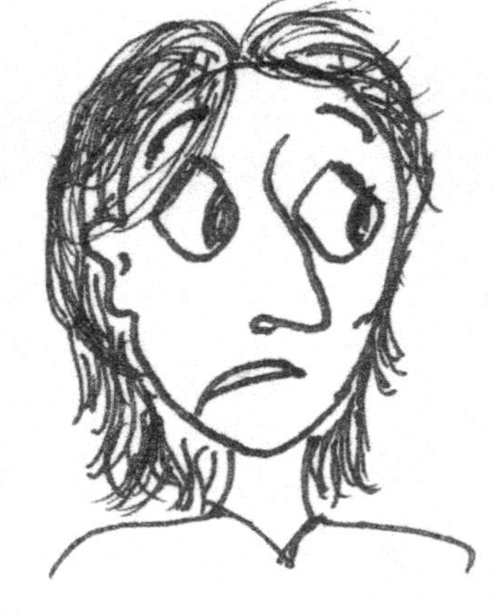

... and you wonder why you cannot do well at work, school & life.

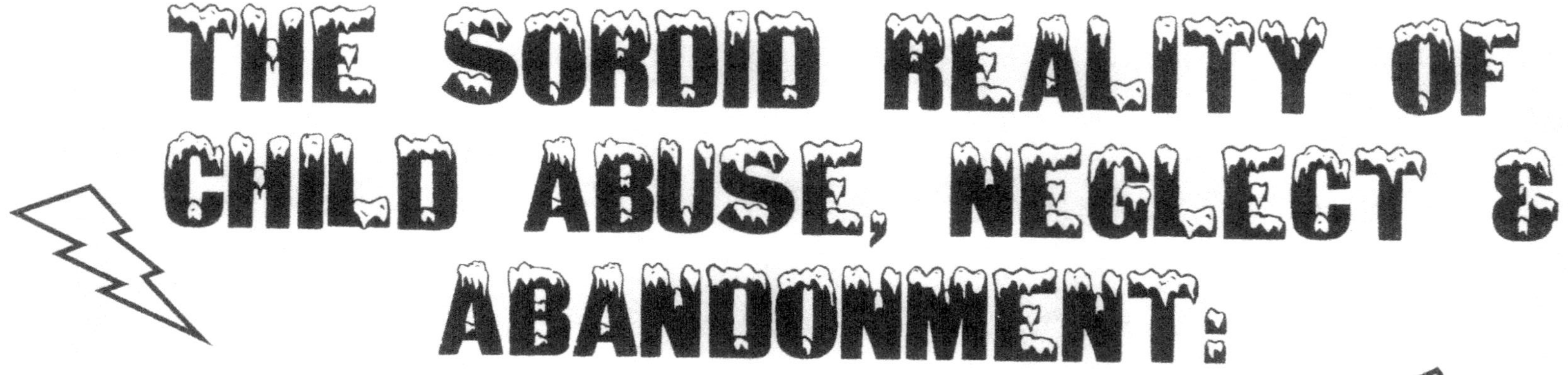

THE SORDID REALITY OF CHILD ABUSE, NEGLECT & ABANDONMENT:

1 in 3 children will experience some form of child abuse;

1 in 4 girls & 1 in 5 boys will experience sexual abuse;

Of those who were sexually abused: 10% were under the age of 5; 35% were under the age of 11; the average age of onset was 7

The vast majority experience multiple abuse experiences; many of them for years

It is estimated that at least 10% of all children have experienced the trifecta: they experience ALL three forms of child abuse, neglect & abandonment

Most of the 'monsters' in our world are NOT the pedophile or rapist, however horrible these events may be.

98% of our monsters live in our homes...

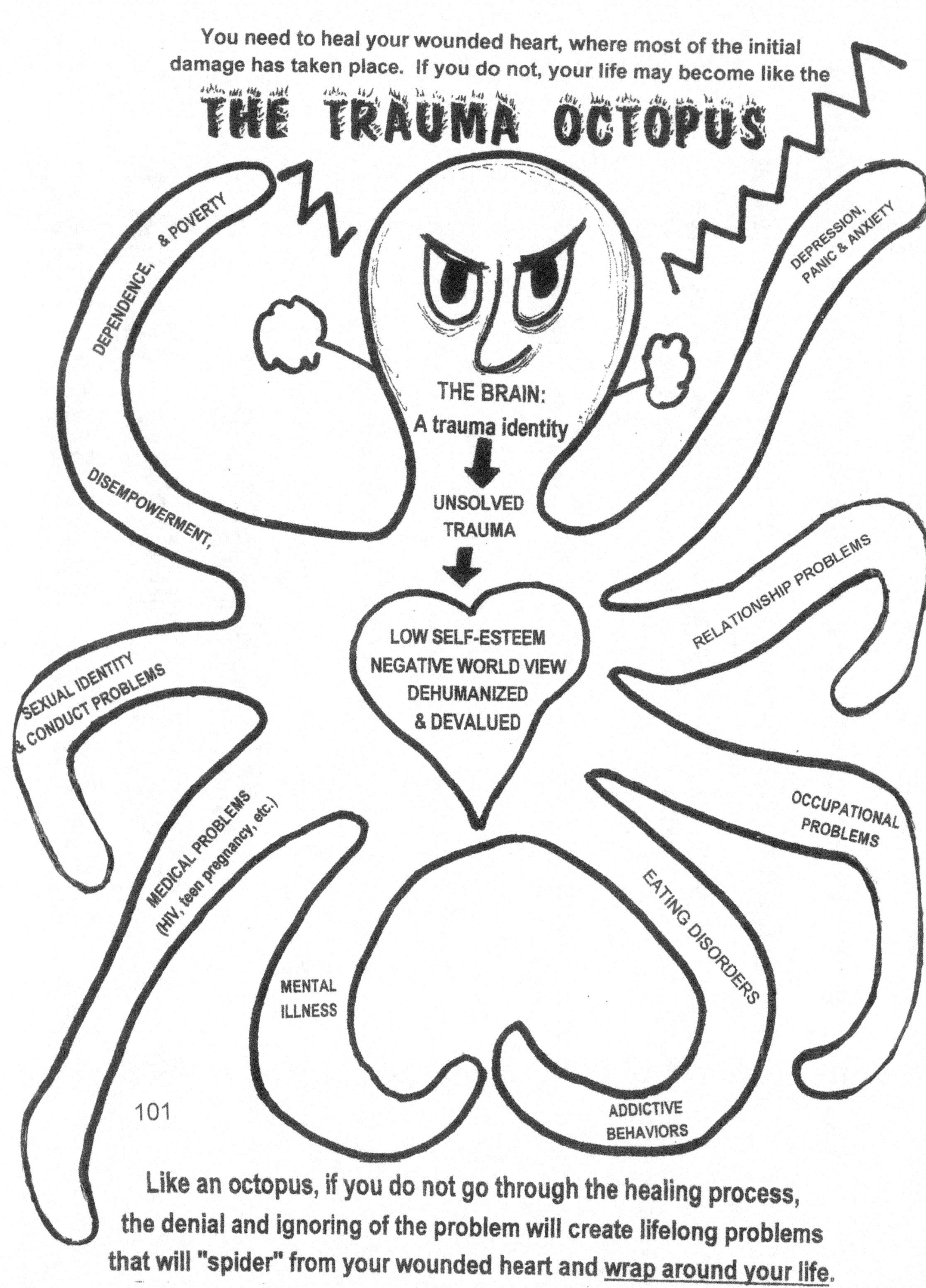
You need to heal your wounded heart, where most of the initial damage has taken place. If you do not, your life may become like the
THE TRAUMA OCTOPUS
THE BRAIN:
A trauma identity
UNSOLVED
TRAUMA
LOW SELF-ESTEEM
NEGATIVE WORLD VIEW
DEHUMANIZED
& DEVALUED
DEPENDENCE, & POVERTY
DISEMPOWERMENT,
DEPRESSION, PANIC & ANXIETY
RELATIONSHIP PROBLEMS
SEXUAL IDENTITY & CONDUCT PROBLEMS
MEDICAL PROBLEMS (HIV, teen pregnancy, etc.)
OCCUPATIONAL PROBLEMS
EATING DISORDERS
MENTAL ILLNESS
ADDICTIVE BEHAVIORS
Like an octopus, if you do not go through the healing process, the denial and ignoring of the problem will create lifelong problems that will "spider" from your wounded heart and wrap around your life.

The Trauma Octopus

"This model is used to show how too many of us CSA survivor's carry the stigma associated with multiple symptoms, at-risk behaviors and lifestyles, and/or socio-economic problems. Too often, these can be a direct consequence of the weakened foundation of one's personality. A child's personality, self-esteem and world-view are usually damaged through the abuse. The betrayal of love and trust, commonly committed by one's own family or friends, can leave a child vulnerable to an array of life's problems, including those listed on the arms of the octopus. As you can see, too many of us survivors share too many of these symptoms.

The model also illustrates how many of us have received treatment or assistance for the symptoms only, without dealing with the trauma issues. This results in temporary relief. We are too often vulnerable to repeat a destructive pattern, or find a new one to engage in. This may not be the fault of the therapists or providers: too often the presenting problem does not touch upon the underlying childhood trauma that may have originated their problems. Therefore, these treatment measures do not reach our BRAINS and our HEARTS (of the octopus), or the foundation of the trauma identity we can develop.

explanation for: The Trauma Octopus, cont'd.

Notice the BRAIN, or the central source of configuring what happens to many of us when we were abused: we may take on a 'trauma identity' or a weakened soul.

Because of this basic weakness and damage committed to a disbelieving child, the results are 'wounded hearts'. This can be demonstrated through: devastating low self-esteem, a world view that 'sees' the world as hostile, hurtful and distrustful; and a dehumanized spirit. This may all leave some of us out of tune with others and a belief that we are devalued: unimportant, insignificant, disgraced, and shameful.

Until our minds and hearts can mend, too many of us simply 're-grow' new octopus arms and continue the self-perpetuation of a negative life and engulfed with a long list of mental health symptoms.

We must help each other 'heal' our wounded hearts to find real recovery and personal empowerment.

Together, HEALING HEARTS!"

Part of this information on the effects of trauma was taken from:

Van der Kolk, Besser, *Traumatic Stress: The Effects of Overwhelming Experience on Mind, Body and Society*, 1996

THE TRAUMA CYCLE

"Around and around: do you get off the merry-go-round or stay hopelessly in pain?"

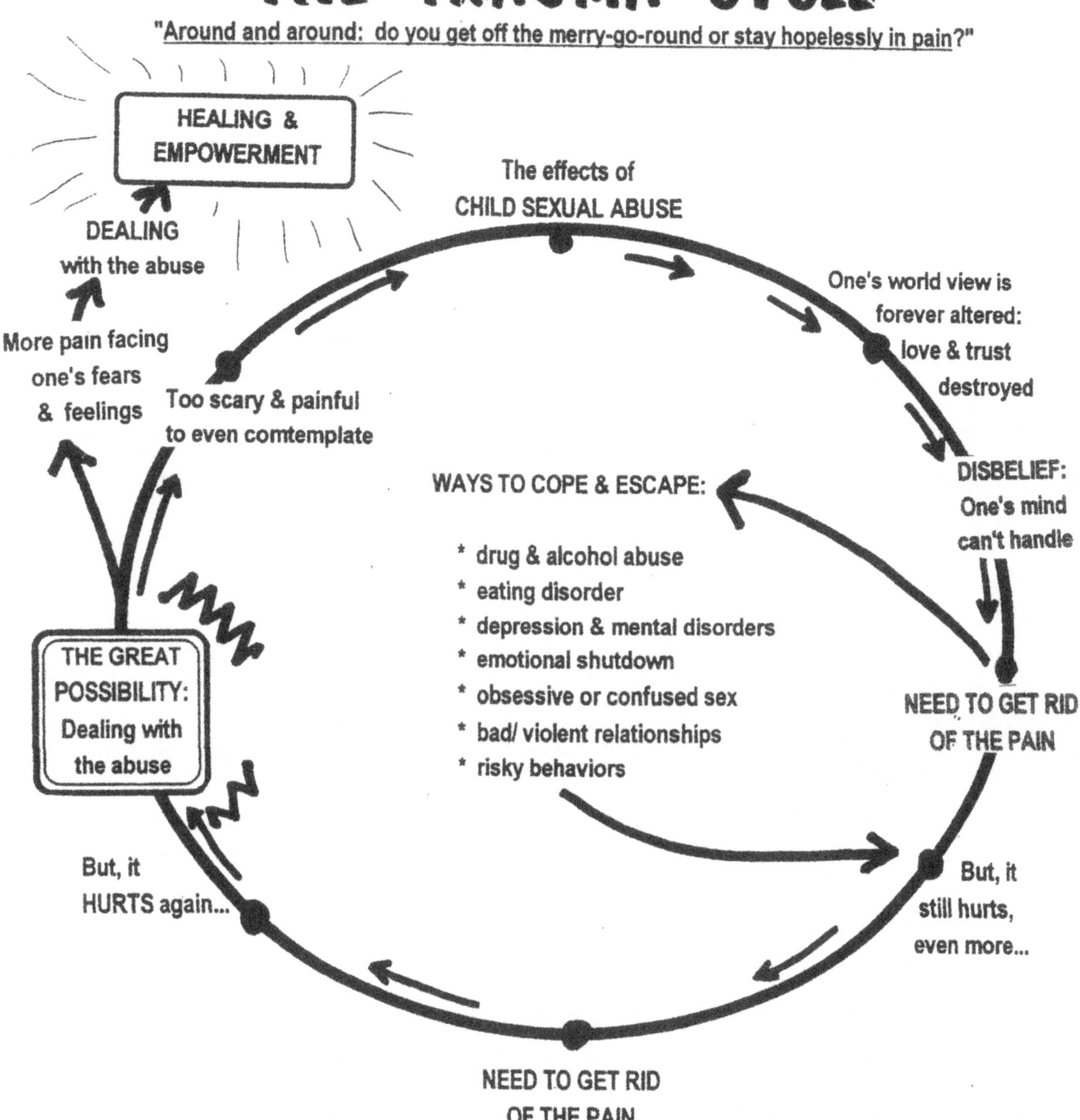

"Why so many survivors repeat the problems of their lives over and over again without resolution or healing."

The Trauma Cycle

These steps would predictably occur with many survivors:

#1: These are all the effects as illustrated on the trauma octopus. this step also includes the awareness that something is wrong and that the sexual abuse is key to a survivor's problems.

#2: CSA (childhood sexual abuse) is devastating to a developing life.

#3: CSA is the ultimate betrayal: a child's whole world is turned inside out. The beliefs of love, trust and comfort, which should be natural entitlements, are all messed up. How does a mind cope with that which should be assumed to be the birth right of all children, and in this case, is not?

#4: As a natural consequence, the mind fulfills its biological reaction to rid the child of the overwhelming pain. ALL humans are equipped with the same defense mechanisms to protect the injured person. This is called the "fight or flight" response: either a person fights to end the pain or if it is too severe, runs away to relieve the mind and/or body of the stress.

#5: A young child can do neither fight or flight- except in the mind (dissociate or repress, for example) or through ways to self-medicate to escape the horrible pain, such as through other substances (alcohol and drugs) or through exerting control (as through risky behaviors and violence). Mental illnesses are often the result of these attempts to cope, which at first, are NATURAL and NORMAL ways to try to adapt to the inadaptable.

(The steps of the trauma cycle, cont'd...)

#6: Unfortunately, their attempts to rid them of unbearable pain, they start producing their own set of negative consequences- and STILL the traumatized person is in pain, usually with more pain.

#7: The cycle continues, with the biological need to get rid of the pain.

#8: The survivor, now often an adult, is now at a major crossroads: do they dive in again to succumb to another round of negative coping mechanisms, quit one destructive choice and start up with another one, or, choose to stand as a warrior and fight the childhood traumatization, still rearing its ugly and devastating stranglehold on the survivor's life.

#9: Unfortunately, in order to really deal with the abuse and end its stranglehold, a survivor most likely will have to endure a period of time of increased stress, anxiety, flooding of emotions, or other PTSD symptoms (post traumatic stress disorder). Expressing feelings and labeling the pain for what it is, vocalizing the story, releasing guilt and shame is once again reliving being that traumatized, vulnerable child. But, if a survivor can endure this temporary pain, believe recovery is possible, receive proper therapy and all the support from other survivors and family that is possible, a survivor CAN succeed. The story and the pain can now be processed and rewritten for what it always was- even if a survivor does not believe it: a violation of your soul without ANY BLAME OF YOUR OWN.

#10: The choice is up to the survivor: does she stay on the merry-go-round and continue self-destructive ways, or get off, endure a period of increased pain, BUT deal with it, and enable oneself to heal, recover, and move into the wonderful world of personal empowerment! THE CHOICE IS YOURS!

★

DO YOU NEED MORE CONVINCING THAT CHILD ABUSE, NEGLECT AND ABANDONMENT CAN CREATE LIFELONG PROBLEMS?

Can you correctly identify what percentage of adult SOCIAL ILLS will occur from the negative effects from unattended childhood TRAUMA some time or another in their lives?

_______ 1. Poverty
_______ 2. Depression
_______ 3. Domestic violence
_______ 4. Incarceration
_______ 5. Sexual problems
_______ 6. Increased illnesses
_______ 7. Drug & Alcohol abuse
_______ 8. School failure
_______ 9. Work failure
_______ 10. Relationship problems
_______ 11. Mental illness
_______ 12. Suicide
_______ 13. Early pregnancy
_______ 14. Anxiety & Panic attacks
_______ 15. Dysfunctional families
_______ 16. Perpetrators
_______ 17. Promiscuity
_______ 18. Aggression
_______ 19. Mistrust of others
_______ 20. Loneliness
_______ 21. Negative world view
_______ 22. Victimhood
_______ 23. PTSD
_______ 24. Phobias
_______ 25. Dead-end life
_______ 26. Low self-esteem
_______ 27. Early death
_______ 28. Loss of dreams
_______ 29. Helplessness
_______ 30. Hopelessness

(These are all proven by research...)

ANSWERS TO:

"Do You Need More Convincing?"

1. 75%
2. 98%
3. 70%
4. 70%
5. 70%
6. 90%
7. 80%
8. 70%
9. 60%
10. 90%
11. 90%
12. 50%
13. 65%
14. 60%
15. 90%
16. 30%
17. 70%
18. 50%
19. 95% +++
20. 60%
21. 80%
22. 70%
23. 50%
24. 40%
25. 60%
26. 95% +++
27. 70%
28. 80% +++
29. 70%
30. 70%

The average is approximately 70% of those who suffer from such afflictions are survivors of child abuse, neglect and/or abandonment

STATISTICS about child abuse, neglect, and/or abandonment come primarily from:

U.S. Department of Health & Human Services &

U.S. Department of Justice

"Most woman have not even been able to touch their anger except to drive it in like a rusted nail."

-Adrienne Rich, Poet

Girls are still socialized not to fight back: it is easier to be hurt and humiliated. To be passive is more socially acceptable than being aggressive or violent towards others- even to stand up for themselves.

Men usually act out their pain...

Women instead act out by acting in.

Thus, self-mutilation techniques, including compulsive overeating, fits the bill of "acting in."

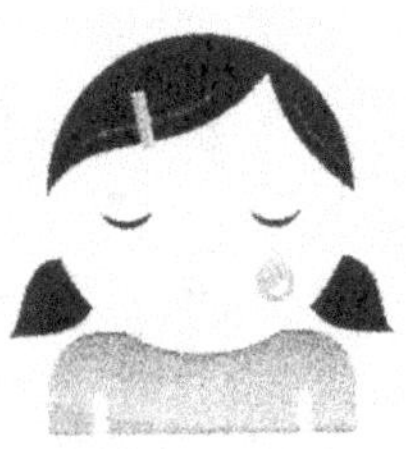

Involving yourself . . .

Do you act out or act in your feelings? ____________________

Which ever way you answered, how do you act? ________________

____

____

____

____

BODY-ARMOUR:

Keep 'em away from your heart by building walls to hide behind...

Although many people are overweight as a result of the common American diet and lifestyle, a large number of survivors are found among the significantly overweight and obese. It's as if layers of fat have been added as a protection against unwanted physical touch. Survivors are generally unsuccessful in dieting and weight reduction programs or quickly regain any lost weight because they feel too vulnerable without the body armour.

Fat is regarded as a sexual turn off, so it protects the victim so it gives the appearance of protecting oneself. Fat is insulation. It's as if you build a fence around yourself.

"You don't know when you feel empty or hungry. You eat to fill up. You eat to feel full. You repress anger and eat to cover it up."

For long term success, survivors must address their issues of child abuse, especially sexual abuse.

Body armour keeps the actual lovers out so the survivor is "free" to "love" oneself...

Food becomes the survivor's main relationship.

Nonessential eating can serve as a substitute gratification alleviating loneliness and bearing a close relationship to human attachment, anxiety and depression...

Involving yourself . . .

Do you feel you developed body armour?

Can you understand how food can serve as a relationship?

The worst damage of obesity is not physical. It's how you ravage any degree of self-worth you have...

Yes, with every chip or candy bar you compulsively eat, you are assaulting your self-esteem and confirming the message of "I'm no good" OR "I'm defective."

"Being fat was my friend. I both loathed it- and wanted it to stay- to keep me safe. This way I was in control. I could reject people (men?) before they rejected me. People couldn't like me any less than I disliked myself.

It kept me from changing- the fear of actually being thin and then exposing my innards, or my true self for all to see- or so I thought.

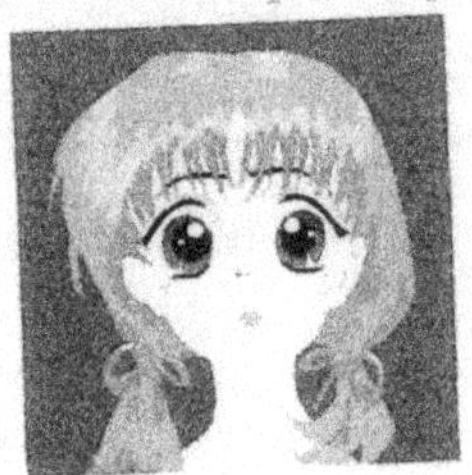

Yes, on one hand I could stay fat and continue my barrage of self-hatred and self-doubt. I could also remain safe: no man could "get me" and my radar for stunningly bad relationships was turned off- just as the men I feared were turned off with my fat. Real or imagined. If they did step into my inner circle if only for a moment, my negative self-talk could chop them all apart and soon they would scoot off into the sunset. Presto! Safe again!

But miserable. Because I wasn't thin, whereas I would supposedly be so "perfect" (right!)

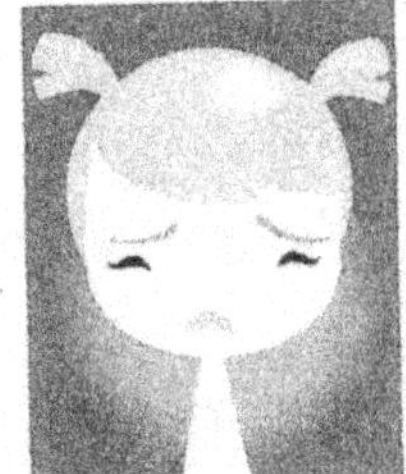

Involving yourself . . .

How would you describe your feelings of self-worth?

Do you believe your feelings of low self-esteem stem at least in part from your abuse experience? ______ If so, in what ways? _________

____

____

Staying heavy- fat! – is a kind of approval for the abuse I had suffered through; for any abuse I may have continued to suffer; and a way to agree with those who would say I cannot be all I am capable of being.

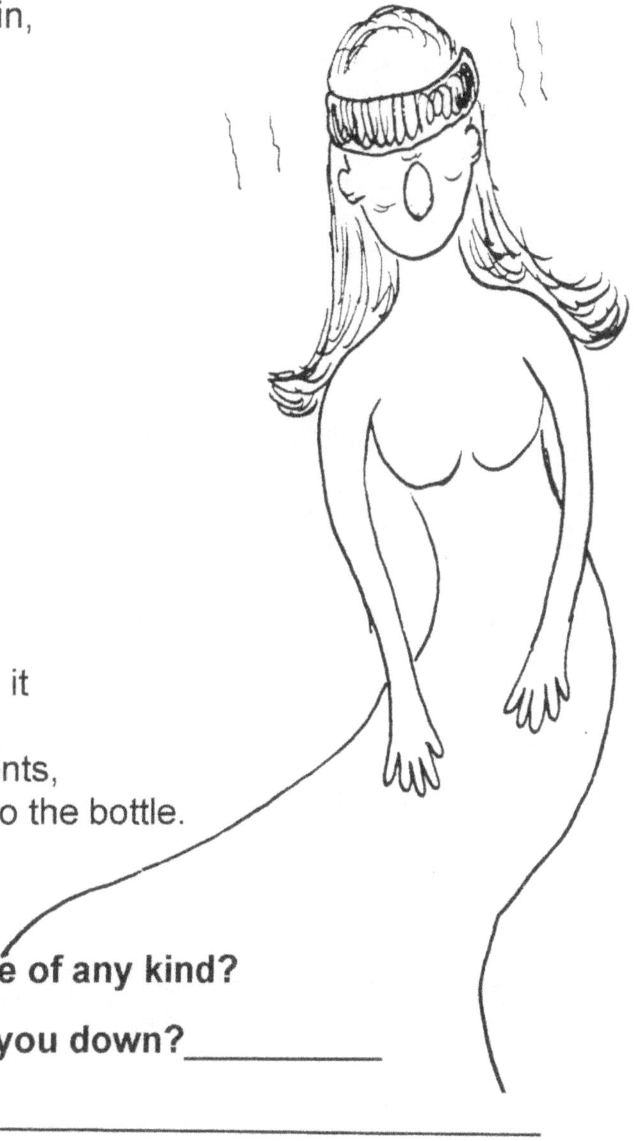

"When I overeat I no longer feel the pain,

Therefore it is softly,
a suspension of any harmful beliefs.

During the eating time,
I am not defective,
I am free!

We all like to escape from time
to time
When life's stressors and troubles
come tumbling along.
But tomorrow,
the healthy work the problems out.

Me,
as a compulsive eater did not deal with it
The next day,
but I ate at those decisive moments,
Like a drunk who cannot stop running to the bottle.

Involving yourself . . .

Do you continue to experience abuse of any kind?

Have you allowed someone to keep you down?__________

If so, in what ways? ____

____

The Road to losing your emotional balance (dys-regulation) as a result of trauma, follows a predictable path:

You experience trauma or abuse

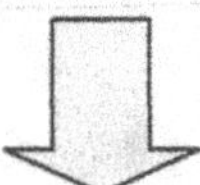

Your brain's amygdala, or early warning system, checks out your response to this trauma experiences

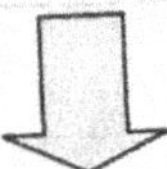

Fight, flight or freeze responses kick in

Your "human" brain cannot respond fast enough to the trauma

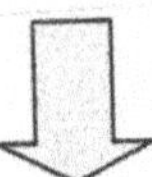

If the trauma is overwhelming, your brain's regulatory system is disrupted

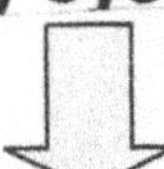

Since thinking is bypassed, you are unable to fully process the trauma

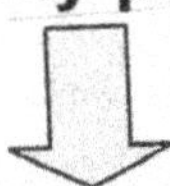

Because of this sloppy processing, things that happen TODAY may trigger emotional responses associated with past trauma, even decades later

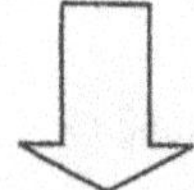

A pattern of recreating, reliving & re-experiencing emotions & actions associated with the trauma begin

More predictable pathways . . .

You often struggle for emotional self-soothing & balance

⇩

When your emotional functioning is disrupted,
it affects your relationships to yourself & others

⇩

You are then left unprotected against a potential wave
of overwhelming feelings. These undigested or frozen feelings
play out negatively time after time

⇩

You may then turn to some addictive substances to self-soothe
& to further perpetuate the destructive trauma reenactment cycle

⇩

SOME SURVIVORS TURN TO OVEREATING
& EVENTUALLY FIND THEMSELVES OBESE

INVOLVING YOURSELF . . .

Which of these steps do you see yourself? ______________________

____

____

____

____

____

____

You're not fighting the Devil of urges, you're trying to stop your feelings from being felt . . .

Some obese people are not able to tell the difference between being scared, angry, and hungry, and so, lump all those feeling together as signifying hunger, which leads them to overeat whenever they feel upset.

Most children learn to distinguish among their sensations, to tell if they're feeling bored, angry, depressed, or hungry- it's a basic part of emotional learning. But girls who have been abused, especially sexually, have trouble distinguishing among their most basic feelings.

They may not be sure whether they're angry, or anxious, or depressed- they just experience a diffuse emotional storm that they do not know how to deal with effectively. Instead you learn to make yourself feel better by eating, that can become a strongly entrenched emotional habit.

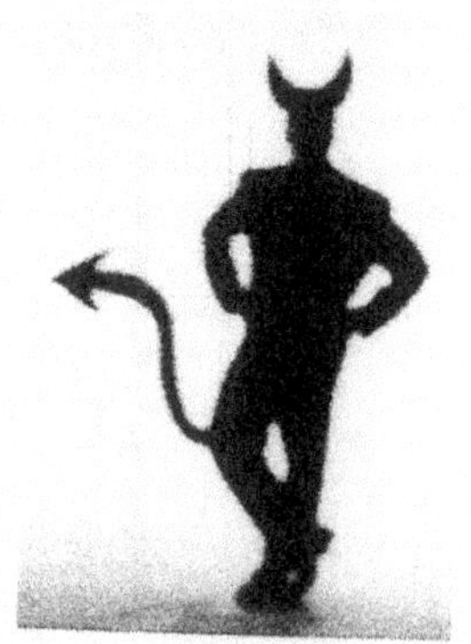

But when this habit for soothing yourself interacts with the pressures you feel to be thin, the way is paved for eating disorders.

"I never touched the bottom of my pain. I became an overeater instead, and in so doing, I EXCHANGED THE NORMAL PAINS OF LIVING; OF BEING ALIVE, FOR THE PAIN OF MY COMPULSION."

Involving yourself . . .

How does this describe you in any way? ______________________________

____

FOOD
(especially goodies!)
is a great way to self-medicate your inner pain.

Do you eat to get full or eat until you're satisfied? Or is that why you never feel full because you're never satisfied?

If you eat in front of the TV or in your car, you can pretend and not take responsibility for and what you're doing.

If you can eat in the middle of a tense conversation, the feelings go in along with the food. You swallow your anxiety and troubled feelings. You get full- but you are left empty emotionally.

I ate for every emotion I felt: when sad, when glad, when mad. Any of them. I used food to glue my life together between hungers.

Food becomes the treasure- even if I did not deserve it. To become hungry is to feel empty- or hollow- that which I based my escape plan. This nonphysical hunger is of the mind, not the body.

and more threatening. And they don't go away just because you fear them...

<u>Involving yourself</u>. . .

Have you ever used food to satisfy your emotional hunger? ________

____

Cookies Wash Away the Pain

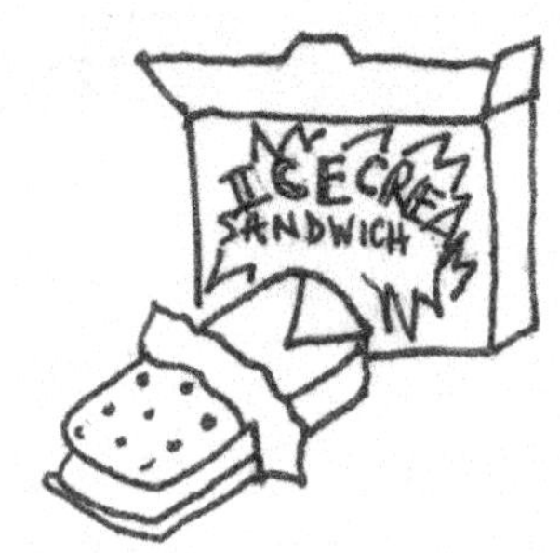

Just one more chocolate chip
and your feelings can leap
out your body's pores
they rapidly seep.
More! More!
You numb your very skin,
you start to believe in life, you'll never win…

Just one more candy bar
and your feelings lick away
up through your head
Oh, now they're gone!
You'll stop this another day
You're here to say
(believe you, right?)
You can make a right with another wrong
(believe me, right?)
You can just write a song called,
"It's just one piece!"

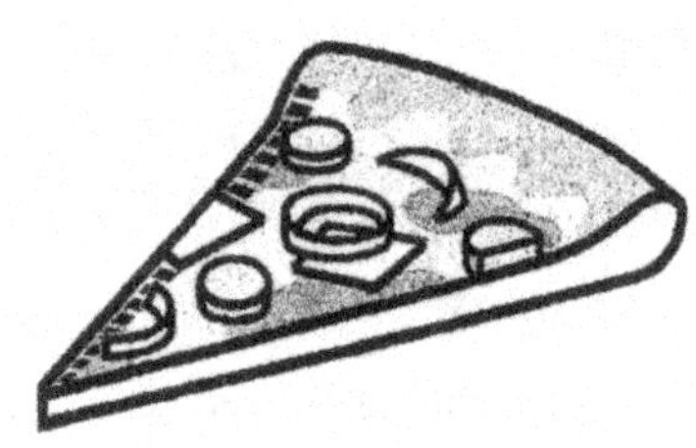

Just another piece of pizza.
Now you're really in the game,
you're never to blame
(but a great feeling buster)
and you can now gleefully say,
No brain, no pain!
More? More?
As you stuff your cheeks
you'll go numb
then call yourself a bum.

When you've downed your last soda pop,
and gorged your other slop
depression warfs over you
like the fog creeping in your space.
In the mirror,
it's you you'll have to face.
But the brow-beating begins
again
"What a slob!"
"What a worthless pig!"
enough assault on yourself like being stoned
for adultery.
Oh, but what the heck!
Throw me another cookie-
you'll forget after that!

The movement from sadness and anxiety to food is fluid and fast

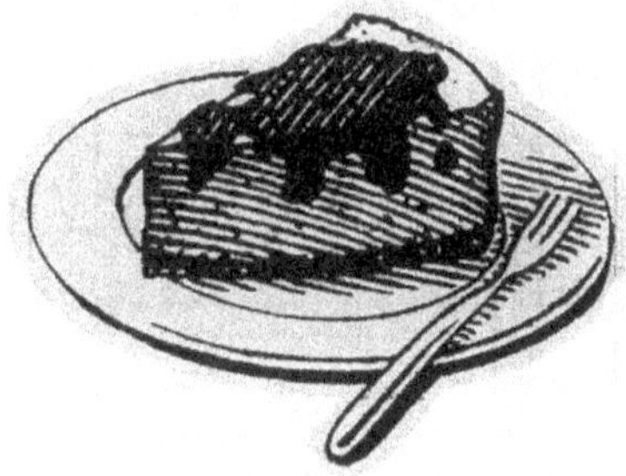

Involving yourself . . .

How do you relate to this poem? ______________________________
____
____

Can you identify with the last statement below the poem?________
____
____

Food was a perfect weapon to attack and rip apart my feelings of self-worth.

Binges are purposeful- but often, subconscious- acts to care for yourself when you do not feel very care for.

Binges are a signal- a sort of red light brightly stressing something is terribly wrong; that you have an unquieted **ache that hasn't been fulfilled.**

Symbolically, you feared others would see what you ate, then "know" you are fat, so then they would not love me anymore.

Everybody eats compulsively from time to time. We all eat too much at Christmas, watching the Super Bowl, or at the county fair. But most people do not beat themselves for days afterwards, like a compulsive overeater does to "punish" themselves to cover up their imperfections.

"If I had been touched and cuddled and held after my abuse, I might not have felt so empty and then symbolically eaten to fill up the emptiness. But because I was "bad" and had "invited" my initial abuse, I could not seek this love because I would then have to admit my wrongness.

Involving yourself . . .

Has food been a weapon for you to attack your self-worth? __________

If so, explain how: ____

____

Were you "touched and cuddled" or otherwise consoled- after your abuse? ____________ If not, how did that make you feel? ____________

____

Oh,
there is an ache
deep inside chasms of pain.
It rains
down on my soul
Deep inside the longing,
the longing
of belonging to more.
To be connected
instead of neglected.

This ache
This ache
this awareness
of the bareness of my feelings
towards all past lovers
But dripping profusely
for you.
I am so blue
when I think of fixing
that which my deeds have corrupted.

So deeply
So deeply
my hopefulness fades
and fades
under the weight of contemplating
the difficulty of relating
to you.
So blue.

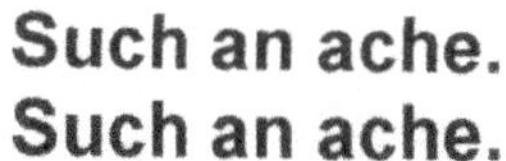

Such an ache.
Such an ache.

Involving yourself . . .

Do you have similar aches in your heart? _________ If so, explain:

___

My compulsive overeating:

A 5-legged response to my child sexual abuse.

The primary drive is to gain the control lost during the abuse.

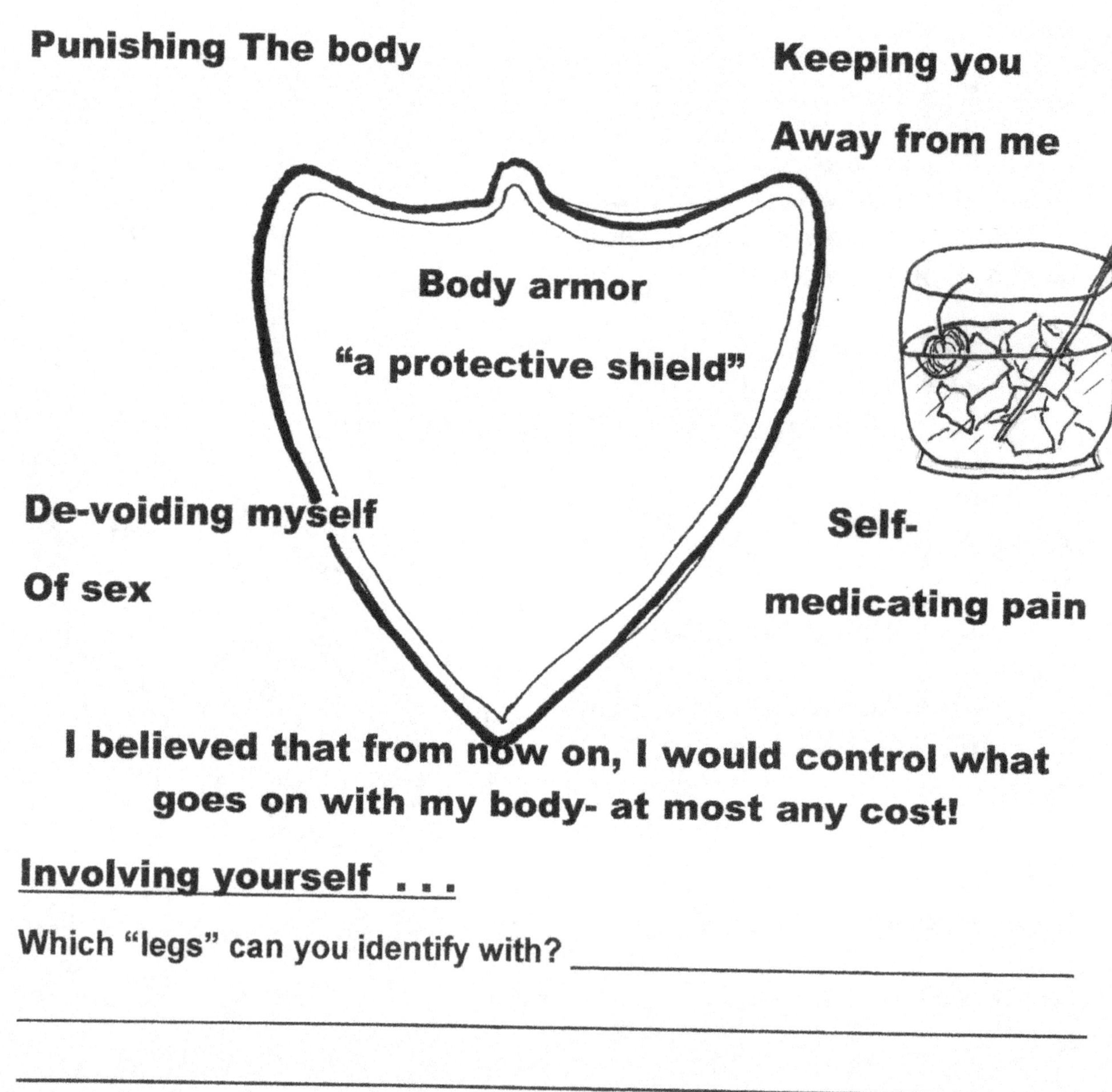

I believed that from now on, I would control what goes on with my body- at most any cost!

<u>Involving yourself . . .</u>

Which "legs" can you identify with? ______________________________

____

____

YOUR response to child sexual abuse:

(1) How do/ did you punish your body? ________________________

____

____

(2) How do you "wear" body armor? ________________________

____

(3) How do you use food to keep others away from your heart?

____

____

(4) How have you devalued your sexuality? ________________________

____

____

(5) How do you self-medicate through food? ________________________

____

____

(6) How much is self-control important to your life? ________________

____

____

When you have a hole in your soul, it is so easy to use food to try and fill it up. So I ate gluttonessly with the foolish belief that if I ate the whole bag of chips or a whole king size candy bar, I would fill up the hole. I was still left with the sad feeling of never getting enough . . .

If I stayed fat, I could look in the mirror and proclaim, "I don't know you! Who is that fat woman?" But before I could answer, when the feelings started to scratch at my door, I'd reach for the popcorn.

SAFE AGAIN!!!

Then a timid question would push up through the fat on my thighs: "What if I discover that my fat was actually helping me so much- to keep my secrets and my secret self- that I just couldn't- or wouldn't- let it go??"

Getting thinner would leave me vulnerable and open to future wounds from future lovers and this scared me to death: I just did not trust in my ability to avoid men who would hurt me. I seemed to be drawn to them- unknowingly- like flies to the fly paper. Because this would be all I deserve, right? Thus, losing weight would be very threatening to me.

To me, this was self-preservation, to keep me "together" even if the "glue" was my fat...

Involving yourself . . .

How do you identify with this narrative? ____________________

____

Do you have a hole in your soul? ________ **If so, describe yours:**

____

____

Do you get enough of what you need? ____________________

____

Everyday,
it's on my mind: **LOSE WEIGHT!**
STOP EATING SO MUCH!
It almost drives me crazy.

Yes,
everyday I will "see the light" and would
set out to tone it down
and stop the gorging.
Everyday.

But jumping out from behind a buttered croissant,
just at the moment
I felt the strongest
and when I could resist any fortified goodie-
out would jump
and arrive- crushing hopeful moments
was the very reason I overate-
that I would scream out
"I deserve bad things happening to me."

And my strong resolve
would melt and dissolve
with the food jumping back into my mouth
("who could blame me?")

"You will always be bad..."

Involving yourself . . .

Is losing weight on YOUR mind all the time? ________________

Do you ever feel you deserve bad things happening to you? ________

____

____

The self-destructive cycle of addiction with the shame, fear, anger and despair can be seen as an imitation of the trauma and abuse...

Addictions (including self-injurious behaviors) fulfills:

	DO YOU IDENTIFY WITH THESE?
Intense feelings can be numbed or amplified	______________________
Pain & discomfort in the body can be eased	______________________
Overwhelming negative thoughts can be drowned out	______________________
Your desperate spirit can be quieted or ignored	______________________

The addiction (in this case, your overeating) becomes the "abuser". You take in the excess food and the cycle of re-enactment begins again . . .

Why is it so "beneficial" for some survivors to engage in some form(s) of self-injurious behaviors?

(Drug & Alcohol abuse, cutting, compulsive overeating, bad relationships, etc.)

TO PROVIDE A
SENSE OF CONTROL
OVER YOUR BODY

TO ALLEVIATE INNER
RAGE WHEN FEELINGS
CANNOT BE EXPRESSED

TO EXPRESS
SHAME
("I am bad...")

TO PROVIDE BIOCHEMICAL
RELIEF FOR SELF-SOOTHING
THROUGH THE BODY'S
NATURAL REWARD SYSTEM

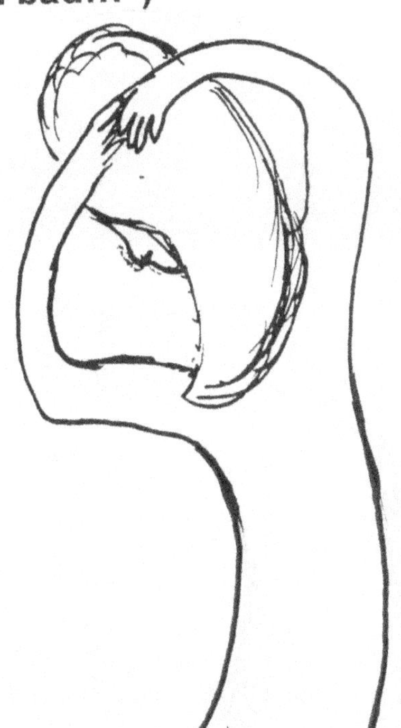

Involving yourself . . .

Which benefits do you get from your overeating?

____

____

____

____

What are the possible functions of YOUR compulsive overeating?

De-scramble the following words to discover the functions:

		Do you use this function?
1. **gleefins**	______________	______________
2. **plenssssheel**	______________	______________
3. **nebeilrol**	______________	______________
4. **romtcof**	______________	______________
5. **tronloc**	______________	______________
6. **seapc**	______________	______________
7. **gasseems**	______________	______________
8. **yeercsc**	______________	______________
9. **divad**	______________	______________
10. **sshitlaprione**	______________	______________
11. **mashe**	______________	______________
12. **bumginn**	______________	______________

FUNCTIONS: *(Use capitalized words for word scramble)*

- A. COMFORT
- B. Avoidance of intimacy or RELATIONSHIPS
- C. To express FEELINGS
- D. To confirm "I am bad…" MESSAGES
- E. REBELLION
- F. NUMBING
- G. Feeding your SHAME
- H. Personal CONTROL
- I. To create SPACE between people
- J. To AVOID feelings
- K. To continue the SECRECY

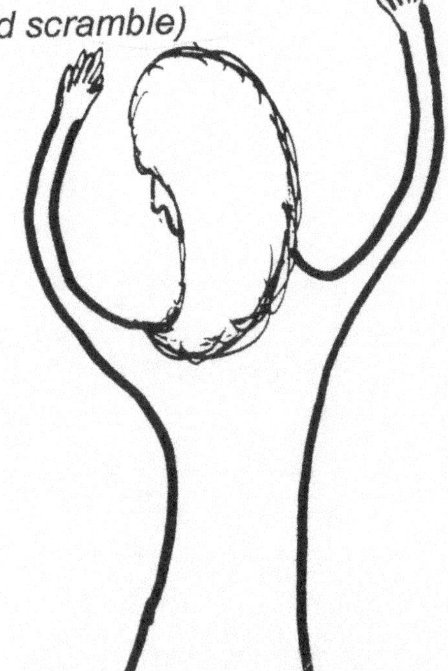

What triggers your compulsive overeating?

TRIGGERING ACTION:	Does this trigger you?
1. depression	________________
2. anxiety	________________
3. societal demands of an Ideal woman	________________
4. low self-esteem	________________
5. family history of overeating	________________
6. co-occurring substance abuse (drug and/or alcohol)	________________
7. media demands	________________
8. feelings of helplessness	________________
9. brain chemistry	________________
10. family dynamics	________________
11. teasing & bullying	________________

For me, as the author,
I have checked off every trigger...

Brick walls, quicksand & other CALLS TO CHANGE I failed to listen to...

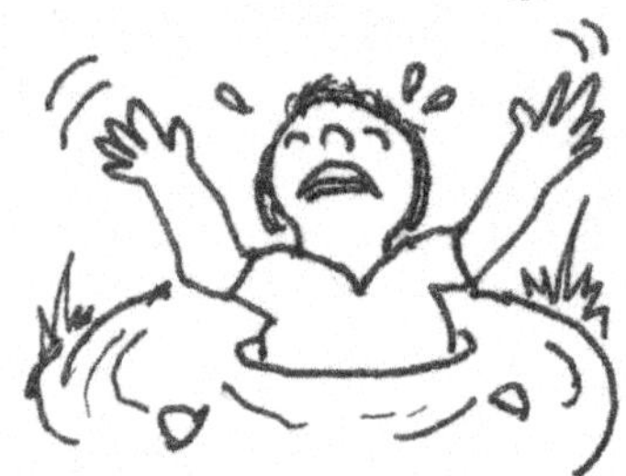

I did not originate the word stubborn, but it perfectly personifies me. How many messages did my body have to tell me before I would really listen? Really listen and then do something about it?

I sure am one to dish out the advice: "do this" or "do that" with all the educational with-it-ness, but ignorance is bliss!

I stand here quite ill- NO! very ill- my body the shelled out battleground. I need to tune in and get with the trek.

No more "What the heck! I will eat it anyways."

NO MORE.

Involving yourself...

Have YOU had enough? ______________ If so, how do you know you are ready for change? ____

____

____

____

The ultimate: SELF-BETRAYAL

28 days.

Not a vampire movie, but a picture from Hell. 11 + 17 days spent in the hospital. Problems with most of my primary organs:

- Lungs which could barely breathe;
- Kidneys which wouldn't flush;
- A heart that beat irregularly;
- and all sorts of other dire health problems.

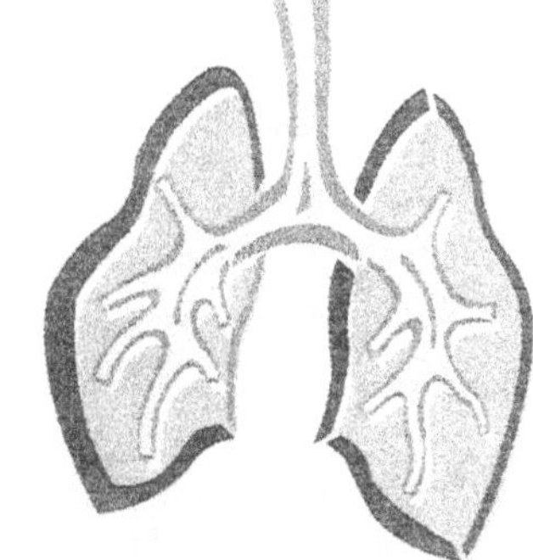

The hospital entrance
equaled the epitome of ignoring the calls to heal.
Healing psychologically could have propelled my physical improvements.

Words screamed out loudly:

There is more than one way to kill yourself...

I almost did succeed, but then I discovered:

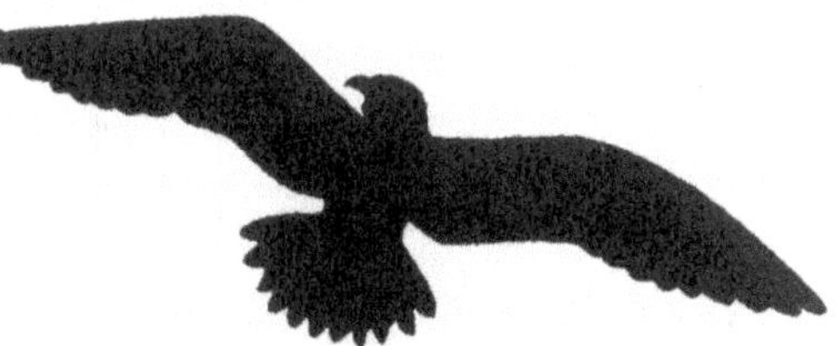

I WANT TO LIVE!

And then I became aware of a growing awareness:

I want to live... my life RIGHT.

Self-betrayal, cont'd...

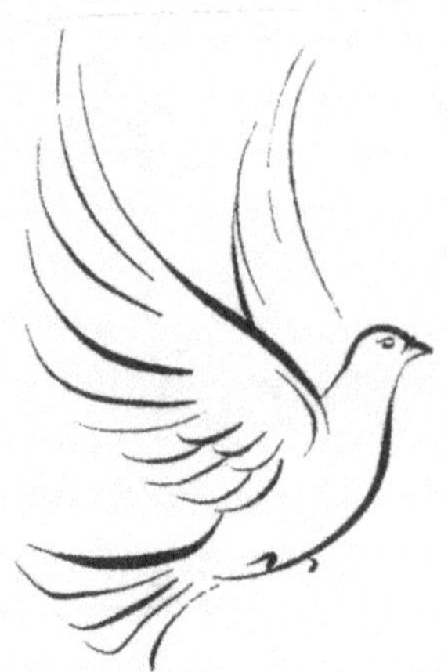

… and my body winced with the strain & pain of it all;
the negative mindset of yesterday challenging still.

But then a major voice smacks me awake and proclaims:

The Best Revenge IS
to Live My Life Right...

... a healing wave washed over me.

Involving yourself...

Proclaim here that you do want to live your life right:

"I, _______________, want to live my life right! I want to become a success in achieving my goals, such as:

____

____

____"

With great predictability, when an overeater is asked if she can see how her abuse past has directly impacted her problems today, even years later, there is often utter denial...

You may say:

"How could what hurt me so many years ago still have a stranglehold on my life today?"

AND

"How could I have surrendered such control to this denial?"

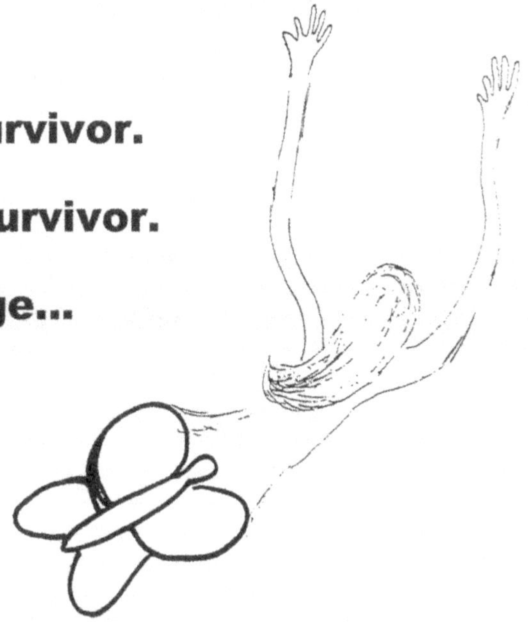

I call me a trauma survivor.

I call YOU a trauma survivor.

It is time to change...

Involving yourself . . .

Do you believe there is a connection of your abuse to some of your significant life's problems? _________ If so, describe how:

____

____

Do you feel it is time for you to change? _______
How will you start?____

____

The Trifecta:
The trauma-addiction-obesity connection

"Your body tells the story of past trauma"
(trauma re-enactment)

It is not enough to merely know who your demon is. You need to discover how it thinks, feels and operates. You need to know how it breathes. Most of all, you need to know how it drove you to want to steer your life so recklessly.

For true healing, you need to resolve your co-occurring trauma (abuse), addiction and obesity issues which have had a stranglehold on your life.

A good mind

In a sea of bad body,

So tired;

So very tired.

So wired in disability.

But can't you see?

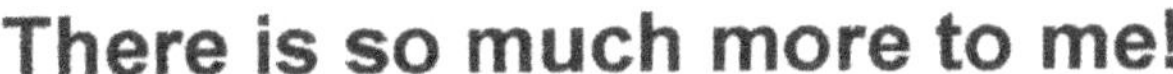

There is so much more to me!

Please look beyond the iris,

Radiating inward.

Notice the soul.

Oh, it is there!!

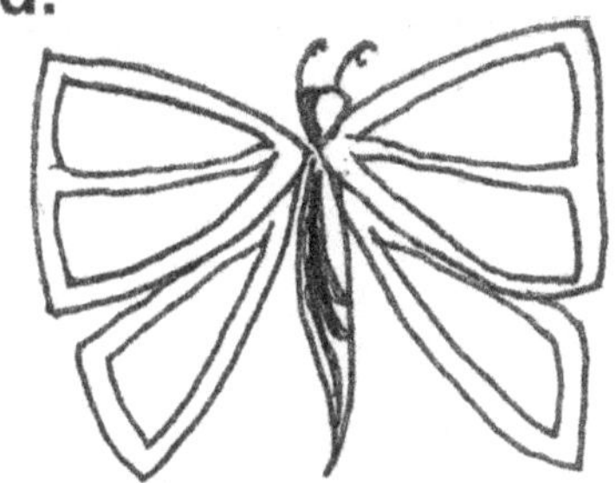

After years of struggling and suffering, my self-loathing and self-sabotaging behaviors have now dissipated into

ACCEPTANCE and PEACE...

The following are the 10 steps for my HEALING JOURNEY. Travel with me...

Now that you have a better understanding of how child abuse (sexual, physical & emotional), neglect and/or abandonment can profoundly contribute to the development of compulsive overeating & obesity, further excavate how these dire childhood crimes spearhead many other social ills such as: mental illness, drug & alcohol abuse, & poverty.

Thereafter, discover what you- or your clients- can do to reverse the damage done through 10 specific healing steps exemplified by the author's own life's story.

The Tears of Wounded Hearts

An in-depth study of how child abuse devastates & too often destroys the newly developing positive self worth of a child through the author's heartfelt confessions as a survivor of child sexual abuse and as a mental health therapist.

Wiping Away the Tears of Wounded Hearts

Offers survivors or clients 10 specific, step-by-step actions for traveling the healing journey in order to soothe wounds inflicted by child abuse and then transform & empower a survivor's life in ways never dreamed of as possible.

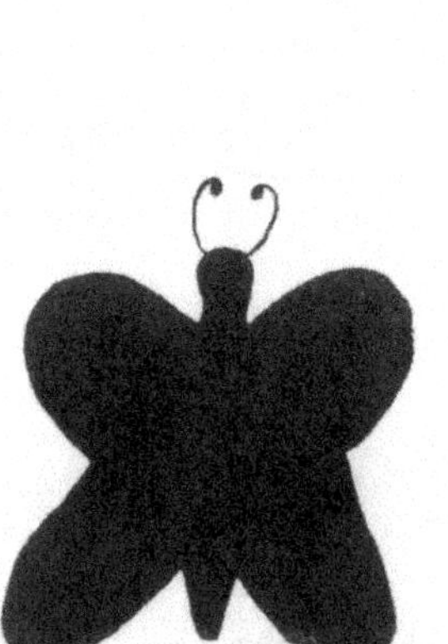

For BOOK ORDER DIRECTIONS, call (716)397-7911 or refer to the front title page.

BIBLIOGRAPHY:

Trauma, Eating Disorders & Self-Injurious Behaviors

Copeland, Mary Ellen, WELLNESS RECOVERY ACTION PLAN, Peach Press, 2002

Ferentz, Lisa, TREATING SELF-DESTRUCTIVE BEHAVIORS IN TRAUMA SURVIVORS: A CLINICIAN'S GUIDE, Routledge/ Taylor, Francis & Bacon, 2012

Harris, Maxine, TRAUMA RECOVERY & EMPOWERMENT, The Free Press, 1998

Herman, Judith, TRAUMA & RECOVERY: THE AFTERMATH OF VIOLENCE, 1997

Kolk, Bessel van de, TRAUMATIC STRESS: THE EFFECTS OF OVERWHELMING EXPERIENCE ON MIND, BODY & SOCIETY, 2006

Miller, Dusty & Laurie Guidry, ADDICTIONS & TRAUMA RECOVERY, W.W. Norton & Co., 2001

Miller, Dusty, WOMEN WHO HURT THEMSELVES, Basic Books, 2005

O'Hanlon, William Hudson, QUICK STEPS TO RESOLVING TRAUMA, 2010

Roth, Geneen, BREAKING FREE FROM COMPULSIVE EATING, Penguin Group, 1984

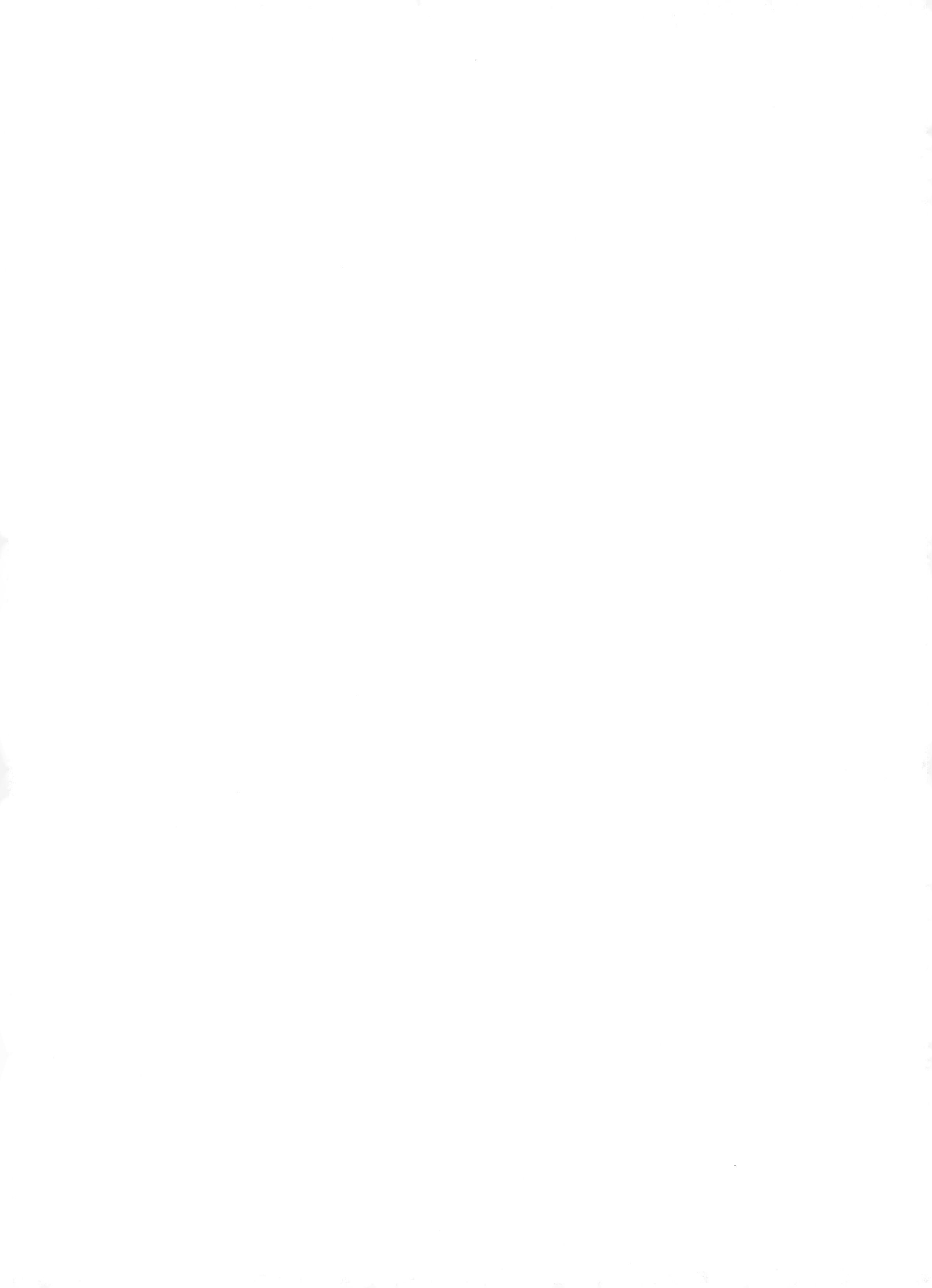

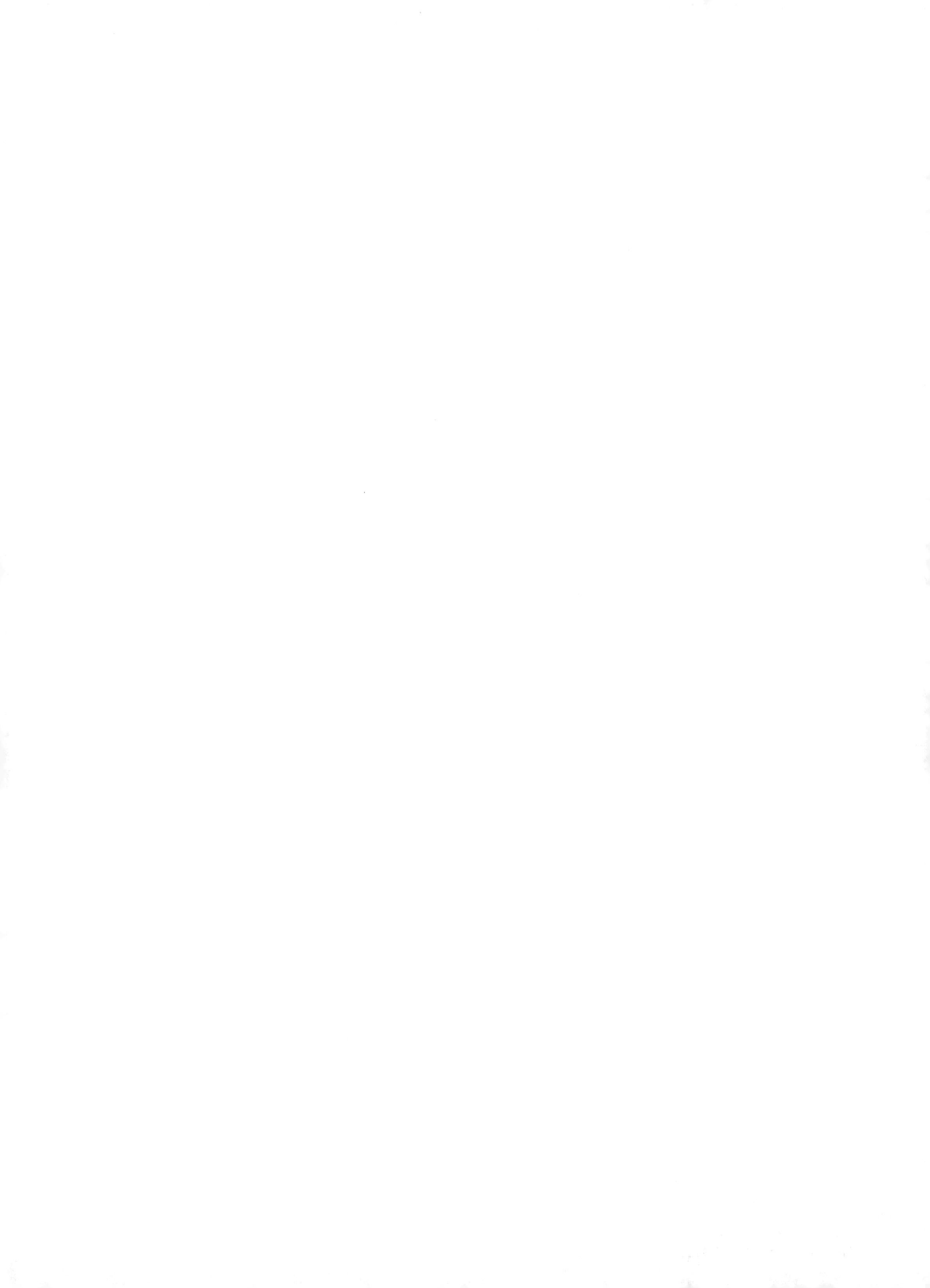

www.ingramcontent.com/pod-product-compliance
Lightning Source LLC
LaVergne TN
LVHW061247100826
845148LV00008B/1052